In That Case

Medical Ethics in Everyday Practice

ALASTAIR V. CAMPBELL
AND
ROGER HIGGS

Darton, Longman & Todd
London
in association with the
Journal of Medical Ethics

First published in 1982 by
Darton, Longman and Todd Ltd
89 Lillie Road, London SW6 1UD

in association with the
Journal of Medical Ethics
Tavistock House North
Tavistock Square
London WC1H 9LG

© 1982 Alastair V. Campbell and Roger Higgs

ISBN 0 232 51557 3

British Library Cataloguing in Publication Data

Campbell, Alastair V.
 In that case.
 1. Medical ethics
 I. Title   II. Higgs, Roger
 174′.2   R724

ISBN 0–232–51557–3

Phototypeset by Input Typesetting Ltd London SW19 8DR
printed in Great Britain by The Anchor Press Ltd
and bound by Wm Brendon & Son Ltd
both of Tiptree, Essex

Contents

Each chapter begins with an episode of the case under study. There are exercises for individual or group work after each chapter.

Preface

Shortly before starting work on this book, one of the authors was shopping with his family on holiday in a small French market town. His son pointed out a disturbing incident at the other end of the street. An elderly man had collapsed, and lay dying on the cobbles. Prodded into action by his son, the wretched author trailed towards the crisis, trying to gather together snatches of suitable French. He found efficient cardiac resuscitation already in progress when he arrived, and he haltingly offered his help.

'Excusez-moi, est-ce-que je peux vous aider? Je suis médecin.'

The resuscitator leaped up with a smile and shook the newcomer warmly by the hand, abandoning healing for hospitality.

'Ah bonjour, monsieur, moi aussi! Où travaillez-vous?'

Discussion while the patient dies may appear to be the hallmark of much medical ethics. Debating professionals sometimes seem to be avoiding, rather than confronting, the real problems, and, in the end, one feels that what really matters to the patient has been forgotten in the excitement of the debate. In this book we try to stay with the patient.

We first worked together on the problem of the practical relevance of medical ethics when we shared the task of planning and publishing the 'Case Conference' series in the newly founded *Journal of Medical Ethics*. This series (and indeed the *Journal* as a whole) aimed to keep all interdisciplinary debate close to actual cases. After six years of such collaboration we were enthusiastic about the thought of a jointly authored book which would present this case-centred approach at greater length. But our experience had not really prepared us for what lay ahead. We had failed to notice the huge distance that lay between a teacher of ethics and a general practitioner, each coming from a radically different area of thought and experience and starting literally, as one colleague remarked, from different premises!

Our attempts to write the book make a minor saga in themselves. We tried working apart, exchanging drafts and writing and re-writing each other's efforts. We tried working together, in our own and friends' houses, in a Highland cottage, in a psychiatric annexe, walking, forever writing fresh drafts, to the resignation of our long-suffering families and the full employment of the local dustmen. Always the answer seemed to elude us. The turning-point came when we discovered Angie. We were led by her tragic story in a way which neither of us had expected. It was almost as if she, not we, were writing the book. She is probably responsible for most of what will be found to be of practical use. What is not must be seen as our poor interpretation of her needs as a patient and a person.

Many other people contributed to our understanding as the book developed – patients, colleagues, students, teachers and friends, too numerous to mention. However, we must single out Bridget Greeves, Rachel Hetherington, Joan and Harold Lambert, Mary Medlicott, Rosalind and David Muston, David Poole, Richard Smith and Ruth Schröck, all of whom gave help and comments which set us right on many points. Janet Prior and Elma Webster typed patiently from draft to draft, with amazing good humour. We owe a very special debt to our families, especially our wives, Sally and Sue. We thank them all, and hope that the readers will now enjoy the reading as much as we have enjoyed the writing.

Alastair Campbell
Roger Higgs

Edinburgh and London, March 1982

Acknowledgements

Thanks are due to the following for permission to reproduce material from copyright sources:

Amber Lane Press: *Whose Life is it Anyway?* by Brian Clark © Amber Lane Productions Ltd.

Faber and Faber for extracts from 'Musée des Beaux Arts' by W. H. Auden from *Collected Poems* and 'This Be the Verse' by Philip Larkin from *High Windows*.

Marvell Press: quotation from 'Deceptions' by Philip Larkin from *The Less Deceived*.

To Angie

I would not dare
Console you if I could. What can be said,
Except that suffering is exact, but where
Desire takes charge, readings will grow erratic?

Philip Larkin 'Deceptions'
The Less Deceived (Marvell 1977)

Introduction

This book is about the everyday moral choices which face people in medical ethics, whether as patients, professionals or members of the society which provides health care. To be of practical use, it must examine real choices. So the book is based on a story, the actual case of a young woman we have called 'Angie Carter'. We have brought the story to life by reconstructing the various episodes in fictional form and we have altered some details to protect confidentiality. In all essential respects, however, the story we tell is a true one and the unhappy events of Angie's life really happened. These events illustrate well the day-to-day issues that may arise when those who are ill seek professional help. Such encounters are a much more important aspect of medical ethics for ordinary people than the extreme and often insoluble dramas which make big headlines. Domestic, unheroic moral issues affect so much more obviously the fabric of our lives, and yet are seldom discussed, either in the news media or in professional training courses.

Words

A problem which faces us at the outset is that the term 'medical ethics' can be a confusing one. To some people it means the special preserve of doctors, where all decisions must be taken by qualified practitioners without outside interference. This is not our view. We believe that other professions and patients themselves may have an equal or even greater part to play in the difficult moral issues which arise from the practice of medicine. Part of the task of medical

1

ethics is to decide which decisions are the responsibility of doctors alone and which should be shared with or passed over to others. 'Medical ethics' is not just ethics for doctors; it is ethics for all those involved in giving and receiving health care.

More confusion arises from the word 'ethics' itself. This can be used in several different senses and at different levels of abstraction. To some, 'ethics' means little more than etiquette, the accepted conventions of a social role. 'Medical ethics' in this sense means correct professional behaviour which is passed on from older to younger practitioners by precept and example. (Some have called this the 'mystical infusion' view!) More commonly, 'ethics' is used as an alternative to 'morals' or 'morality'. Thus we speak of an 'ethical' code or a 'moral' code and of 'unethical' or 'immoral' behaviour. Here 'ethics' refers not just to socially acceptable behaviour but to what is claimed to be good or bad, right or wrong in an objective sense. This is how we shall be using 'medical ethics' in most of our discussion. We shall be asking whether the actions of the people who tried to help Angie were right or wrong, whether the relationships were good or bad, and we shall look for ways in which the quality of such professional relationships can be improved.

There are, however, other uses of the term 'ethics', which are also important for understanding the nature of medical ethics. The academic discipline known as moral philosophy, or ethics, is concerned with the critical study of morality, seeking the fundamental principles, norms or values which lie behind particular moral judgements. At a higher level of abstraction, philosophers discuss the meaning of moral terms like 'good' and 'right' and the relationship between moral reasoning and reasoning in other fields, such as science or aesthetics. We refer only in passing to such abstract questions in this book, not because we regard them as unimportant, but because our aim is somewhat different. We want to encourage the kind of critical attitude to professional practice which is required before the usefulness of the more abstract questioning can be appreciated at all. In this way, our book could be seen as an 'appetizer' for moral philosophy. On the other hand, we do not see a need for every practitioner to study

2

ethics at this abstract level. Our aim will be fulfilled, if people realize that in order to act morally (in professional or in personal life) they need to develop both increased sensitivity and a more self-critical attitude. These are the 'beginnings of wisdom' so far as ethics at any level is concerned.

Method

In order to keep our argument close to practical issues, we have interwoven the discussion of the different aspects of moral decision-making with successive incidents in Angie's life history. We shall see Angie through many different eyes. At times she is the centre of attention; at other times she is 'off stage', yet still an important character. As the story unfolds, certain aspects become clearer, others more obscure. There is never a 'complete picture', for such things exist only in textbooks, not in real life. Our readers will probably find themselves identifying with at least some of the professional helpers in the story as well as with Angie herself or a member of her family. The exercises at the end of each chapter are designed to aid such identification, allowing readers to imagine what they would have done, and to use the Angie story as a starting-point for a wider consideration of the practical and moral issues in health care.

This method inevitably involves some repetition in the arguments of each chapter. The same moral issues reappear with different emphases and in different contexts as the story unfolds. Thus our exposition does not proceed in a linear fashion from premises to conclusion. Instead we circle round the issues, building up a composite picture of moral choices by taking elements which are all present in the first chapter and focusing on them one by one in the succeeding ones. The final chapter recapitulates the whole discussion, and extracts from it practical guidelines for future use.

Readers

Few people are likely to avoid some contact with professional health services during their lifetimes. Thus this book may prove helpful to a wide range of readers. Obviously people

3

working as doctors, nurses, social workers, health visitors, chaplains or para-medical professionals will find themselves directly or indirectly addressed by our discussion of professional ethics. We have written the book with the students of these professions especially in mind and hope that it may prove useful as a basic textbook in a variety of courses. But patients, the relatives of patients and the wider public all feature in our discussion also. A good measure of our success will be the extent to which the book appeals to such a wider readership, without losing its specialized interest for professionals.

It may be that the biggest problem in medical ethics is the gap which exists between those who seek help and those who offer it. Perhaps the story of Angie can help to bridge that gap.

1

Choices

There were a lot of steps up to the flat on the fifth floor. Dr McVie wondered why lifts, even in quite expensive blocks, broke down so often. Since he'd turned fifty, he'd found the architects seemed to design each step a little higher than the one before. He stopped to breathe and think.

From the balcony, autumn mist lay over the city, hiding the big bonfire and the guy in the park at his feet. No facial burns like those two last year, please.

With a jump, he realized he was putting off a visit, and beyond that the start of an evening surgery. What was he going to find at the Carters'? He leafed through his mental files, trying to grasp the essentials.

He had been called to visit Angie Carter, now just 16, who had apparently been off school all day. She was a bright thing, he knew, but an 'only' because Mrs Carter had had 'a bad time' with her, and had later had a mastectomy for breast cancer. Apart from that difficult time he had seen the family seldom as Mrs Carter, rather a tough nut, was a secretary with high standards and a tendency to want to manage minor medical things herself; and he liked that. Mr Carter was a hard-working warehouse foreman with little to bring him to the surgery.

Angie had the strange mixture of rather leggy attractiveness and determined naivety that he remembered in his own second daughter, and he liked to chat with her. All the same, some wordless anxiety had stuck at the back of his mind last time he had seen her, when in spite of a real sore throat he felt she had wanted to talk about something else, but hadn't. Now she had tummy ache, and had been at home all day.

His knock brought a welcome, but not the one he wanted. Mrs Carter showed him through the living room in heavy silence. The atmosphere was alive with tension. Angie lay in bed, staring at the

5

wall, her eyes half closed. She grudgingly gave him details of her pain and he gently examined her. Her tummy was tense, but no surgeon or gynaecologist would be interested. As a father he was very relieved, as a doctor rather disappointed.

'I don't find anything too wrong here. Certainly there's nothing inflamed.'

Pause.

'You seem rather tense, Angie.'

Mrs Carter broke in, unwelcome. 'It's been a terrible time these last few days, Doctor. I was sure it was all nerves, but John insisted I call you, that it was best to be safe. You see, Angie has been going out with a boy, who, well, you know how it is round here, very *mixed*, and well, he just isn't the one for *her*. Angie is all set to get her 'O' levels and get into the Poly, but last week she just ups and announces she's going to leave school and marry her Tony – just like that! John feels it's far too soon and I'm between the devil and the deep when these two begin to fight, and, as you can see, it really has taken its toll on Angie. I know you can't solve all our problems, but can you give her something to calm her down?'

Silence. He hoped Angie would be drawn into words.

'Is that how it is, Angie?' – gently.

No answer, but a large tear rolled down past the mole on her right cheek. The counterpane heaved, the turned-up nose sniffed, but no more. Her blue eyes reflected only on herself. How could he get rid of Mrs Carter, so that Angie could relax?

Monday evening waiting room began to buzz in his head.

He took Angie's hand, then dropped it and reached for his prescription pad. 'Will you take these, and come to see me tomorrow evening?'

No answer. He turned to hand the paper to Mrs Carter. Her relief increased his discomfort. He opened the door back into the living room, which was now full of smoke and Mr Carter. He had been drinking, and was pacing the room.

'Did she tell you? I'm sorry to call you, Doctor, but you know how it is. That little bastard – if she marries him, I've told her, I've told her – it's over my dead body.'

The still evening air outside was a relief.

When Dr McVie climbed the stairs to the Carters' flat he was in a reflective mood, but not one that prepared him for the choices which awaited him. Though a kindly and thoughtful man, he was caught in a routine learned from years of medical practice. He had been in the game long enough to sense something of what was going on in the family, but prescribing pills seemed harmless and released him for the evening surgery ahead. His action broke no obvious rules and offered an immediate practical solution. But did he really act for the best? And could he have chosen otherwise?

For Dr McVie it was just another busy Monday in urban general practice, and decisions to be made – on average, at least one every six minutes, it seems.[1] We may deplore the statistics for the sake of patient or doctor or both, but choices of action are being made at that sort of speed in any place where health problems are brought to a professional worker, whether in hospital or community, central Africa or Stoke Newington. Many of the choices seem to be straightforward professional decisions: Should I do a more extensive examination? Is a specialist opinion called for? How soon should I see this patient again? But other aspects of the choices seem less easy and involve evidence and attitudes which are not always part of a professional training curriculum: Why is the patient not co-operating? How far have I the right to intervene in this family's internal quarrels? Will my treatment do any good? These broader questions may seem a pointless, even dangerous, interruption of professional activity, rather like stopping to check a car's tyre pressures on a journey through rush-hour traffic. Yet tyres do have to be checked at an appropriate time, or a nasty accident could occur. In the same way, the basic assumptions which guide professional decisions and patients' responses to these decisions need regular critical examination or their morality may be of dubious worth.

Most professionals who have to make their own decisions have been brought face to face with the moral issues at some time. Often this was when, as students, they were first confronted with a dying or deeply disturbed patient, or later, when more intimate knowledge of their profession made them doubt its effectiveness. Sometimes it was just over lunch with a friend, or after a TV serial in the evening. But sometimes it was when a sudden crisis erupted – a clash with a patient or colleague, and no time to think. On these occasions, re-

7

sponses tend to be automatic, often beyond immediate conscious control and rarely helpful or illuminating. Afterwards they may wish they had been better prepared for such clashes, but *how* to prepare for them remains a puzzle. It is as though ethics is a kind of minefield, and no one has thought to provide a map.

Of course not everyone would agree that we should even try to prepare ourselves for moral decisions. 'When people start talking about ethics I reach for the golf clubs', remarked one consultant in a case conference. He was reflecting a widely held view that ethics is really a matter of common sense and experience, and that professionals will easily pick it up as they go along. The uncritical nature of this view is no less worrying than its opposite, which asserts that there is a single all-embracing and inerrant ethical system, which should be taught to everyone. The approach of this book is opposed to such simple solutions. We want people to take time out from their routine professional practice in order to reflect on the morality of their actions. We do not think that there are simple and unambiguous answers to the questions which such reflections will raise. But we hope to suggest a number of useful methods for pursuing the questions both alone and in discussion with others.

With these points in mind we return to the situation which Dr McVie encountered when he visited Angie. The four people in the Carters' flat that afternoon each acted in a particular way. Mrs Carter sought to impress the doctor with the seriousness of the situation and the need for him to offer some relief. Angie conveyed by tears and silences the depth of her misery and the uselessness of help. Mr Carter broadcast his agitation in clouds of cigarette smoke and angry words. Dr McVie offered help with well-used instruments: a kindly manner, a reassuring hand and the prescription pad.

If we want to discuss the moral aspects of these actions and interactions we need to assess them in some way. For example, we might ask, was the outcome the best that one could expect from this house call? This question assumes that we judge actions according to the results they achieve. The more useful or beneficial the results, the better the action. Such a view (known to philosophers as utilitarianism) must then offer a criterion for deciding which results are most beneficial. For example, we might assess benefit according to the amount of happiness caused or the amount of pain avoided for all the people involved.[2] So, we could say that the outcome of the house call was a good one, since Mr and Mrs Carter were reassured that Angie was not seriously ill and were given the prescription for her which they wanted; Dr McVie was able to get away from an uncomfortable situation and start his evening surgery; and Angie had access to a drug which would alleviate her anxiety. But as soon as we assess the outcome in this way we are left with doubts. Firstly, we could regard this assessment as too superficial. Will this house call *really* make Angie and her parents happier? Perhaps it has just covered over a conflict which will emerge again later in a worse form. And what about Dr McVie? He may feel relieved at present, but perhaps his conscience will trouble him later for giving in so readily to Mrs Carter's demands. So it could be that the results will, in the long term, cause more unhappiness than happiness. Who can be sure in any situation what the final outcome will be? Defenders of the utilitarian approach to ethics answer this objection by pointing out that we learn from experience what is most likely to promote happiness and on the basis of this work out 'rules of thumb' to guide our actions. Most of the time those rules will get the desired results, but if not then we can change them for other rules which are more effective in promoting general happiness.

But now a second objection may be made. What about the rights of individuals if only general happiness is considered? Let us suppose that the house call benefited Dr McVie, Mrs Carter and Mr Carter, but not Angie. Was the outcome good or bad? If only the benefit of the majority matters then it was good, but many people would argue that the rights of individuals are more important than promoting general happiness.[3] This objection leads to a different way of assessing Dr McVie's house call. We can ask, did Dr McVie and Mr and Mrs Carter act rightly or wrongly in the way they dealt with Angie? This question assumes that there are certain norms or standards for judging the rightness or wrongness of our actions, especially when they affect other people. Frequently these standards are enshrined in moral codes, such as the Ten Commandments. Such codes define certain actions as wrong in themselves (e.g. blasphemy, murder, theft, adultery, lying).

In medical ethics the Hippocratic Oath has been a source of judgements of this type, in relation to euthanasia, abortion, confidentiality and purity of professional life. Modern codes of medical ethics such as the Declaration of Geneva of the World Medical Association follow broadly similar lines, but with less decisiveness on issues like abortion.[4] The difficulty, however, is that such codes often seem far removed from the ordinary issues of daily professional practice. Dr McVie could not be accused of unethical conduct in terms of breaking a specific rule in a professional code, yet somehow the inter-actions between him, Angie and Angie's parents seem unsatisfactory. As so often in daily life, there are no utter villains and no flawless heroes or heroines – just a less than ideal set of relationships between people. Codes of ethics seem too general and abstract to deal with these grey areas.

Therefore, instead of assessing the house call in terms of results or by reference to the rules of an ethical code, we can attempt a third method of assessment. We can ask, what was the nature of the relationship between the various people involved? This third method of assessment will be the dominant one throughout the rest of the book, since we believe it to be the most useful in providing insight into the morality of everyday medical encounters. This is not to deny the usefulness of looking also at codes of ethics and at practical outcomes, but we regard these as secondary to evaluating the nature of the relationships between those seeking help and those offering help in professional health care. It is here that we most urgently need criteria for moral judgement.

Autonomy and Paternalism

What was it about the relationship between the people in the Carters' flat that makes us uneasy? It has something to do with the way in which everyone seemed to be manipulating or attempting to manipulate everyone else. This is obvious in the case of Mrs Carter. She tried hard to control the situation, setting the atmosphere as soon as the doctor arrived and making sure that she got his attention throughout. (The fact that Dr McVie handed the prescription to her is a good measure of her success!) Mr Carter had his own way of making people feel under pressure, and we discover that he was the instigator of the house call and a major source of Angie's anxiety. Angie herself used passivity as a weapon – the sore tummy, the tears, the refusal to talk. (Her parents might take her to water, but they couldn't make her drink!) In this tussle of personalities Dr McVie seemed to feel helpless and inadequate. Abandoning attempts to communicate with Angie, he used his prescription pad as a passport to the freedom of the fresh autumnal air outside.

No one in the flat that afternoon was willing to give Angie her own choice, not even Dr McVie, who prescribed a drug for his patient without obtaining her consent and with no evidence that she had agreed to his suggestion of consulting him privately later. We can therefore describe the actions of the parents and the doctor as 'paternalistic'.[5] They treated Angie as though she were an incompetent child, unable to take responsibility for her own treatment and unable to exercise her right of choice about how this treatment should be administered. The fact that Angie colluded in this paternalism by retreating into a childlike passivity does not justify it. Angie was not a child. Although not yet fully an adult perhaps, she was (in terms of law and of her physical development) perfectly capable of having a sexual relationship with her boyfriend, of leaving the parental home and of getting married, if she wished. Angie, the young woman with difficult choices before her, was completely by-passed by the decision to prescribe a tranquillizer for her tension-related stomach pain, whether she wanted it or not. It is hard to see how this could have contributed to a healthy outcome for her.

The moral objection to such paternalism (and to other forms of manipulation which attempt to limit people's choices) is that it threatens the individual's freedom and dignity. In philosophical terms, it threatens 'autonomy'. Autonomy is the capacity which each person possesses for directing his or her own life according to freely chosen goals or values. Obviously autonomy is not an 'open and shut' matter.

The degree to which people are capable of it varies according to their age, mental capacities, social circumstances and emotional state. In addition, the autonomy of one person is limited (or should be) by the need to respect the autonomy of others. Only a beast or a God (as Aristotle put it)[6] can live as though he were not part of society, with all the limitations on individual freedom which that entails. Nevertheless, any individual has some scope to determine and pursue personal aims. A vital function of morality is to protect and promote such freedom, especially in the vulnerable members of a society, who cannot readily defend themselves against external threats.

Medical encounters contain a specific hazard to autonomy because the sick person is in a weak and dependent position.[7] It is easy for people who offer help to begin to take over the patient's life, feeling that they, from the vantage point of their professional expertise, know best. Dependency as an unwanted side-effect is not just limited to drugs. As we have seen with Angie, patients themselves frequently encourage this attitude by regressing to a childish and over-dependent state, seeking to put responsibility for their recovery on to the shoulders of their professional helpers. From the point of view both of morality and of health enhancement such attitudes may be disastrous. Of course the patient is bound to be dependent on professional help and advice: but this dependence should be a temporary expedient, voluntarily entered into, with the sole aim of restoring freedom and self-direction to the patient. The basic goals of health care – preventing premature death, alleviating pain, overcoming disease and disability, promoting health in individual and society – could all be summarized under the single heading: enhancing autonomy. Unfortunately the means to this goal, which can include a period of diminished freedom and a loss of independence, can obscure the ultimate aim – the return to independent functioning. Recovery is autonomy restored.

Consent and Competence

In view of the hazard of autonomy contained within professional health care, we need to look carefully at the notion of

12

consent, which forms the basis for treatment in virtually all cases.[8] We have already stated that Dr McVie prescribed a drug for Angie without obtaining her consent to treatment. But is this fair to Dr McVie? Had she not given what we might call 'tacit consent'? She had gone to bed, letting her mother call the doctor. She allowed Dr McVie to examine her and answered *some* of his questions at least. When the prescription was offered, she did not say that she was opposed to it. Given her upset emotional state, was this not enough for the doctor to go on?

The ambiguities in Angie's case provide an excellent illustration of the problem of defining what we mean by valid consent. By saying that Angie gave tacit consent we could be suggesting that, provided people do not actively *resist* health care interventions, there is no objection to them. But this is a very dangerous step. It puts the patient into the position of the passive recipient of any treatment which a professional can administer without eliciting a protest. Mere presence in a sick bed, a clinic or a hospital ward would make the patient 'fair game', as it were. Consent must be understood in a much more active sense than this. The professional must be prepared to justify the treatment to the patient – explaining what is to be done, why it is necessary, what its effects will be and whether there are alternative measures which could be taken. The patient must be left free to refuse the treatment, taking responsibility for the consequences of so doing. Anything less than this drastically reduces the voluntary nature of the relationship between patients and professional helpers.

However, in saying that Angie gave tacit consent, we could also be suggesting that she would have co-operated with Dr McVie, had she not been so angry with her parents. Since Dr McVie already knew her, he felt justified, perhaps, in interpreting her silence more as a device to annoy her mother than as a refusal of the treatment he was offering. This takes us into the area of *competence* to give consent. Dr McVie guessed that Angie would have co-operated if she had not been so upset. In other words he regarded her as incompetent to decide for herself at that moment. We must assume that the combined forces of time and Mrs Carter made him act in this way. A safer, though more difficult, solution would have been to ask Mrs Carter to leave, while he tried more persistently to find out how Angie herself felt she could be helped. There are, however, many situations in which the option open to Dr McVie is simply not available. The patient may be unconscious, or severely mentally disturbed, or too young or too mentally retarded to understand adequately. Such patients are clearly incompetent to give consent (though it is important to be flexible in drawing this boundary for any particular patient). In such cases a relative, guardian or appropriate authority must decide whether or not to give consent, attempting the difficult task of choosing what they believe the patient would want or what would be in the patient's best interests.

But such factors did not arise in Angie's case. There was no moral justification for Dr McVie and Mrs Carter to ignore her refusal to co-operate. Upset or not, she was perfectly competent to decide whether she wished to lower her tension and anxiety by taking tranquillizers. No one should have made that choice for her.

Choice and Realism

Yet – when all has been said – it must be admitted that making a choice is far from simple. To say that someone chose a line of action suggests a clear knowledge of alternatives and the conscious selection of one of them. In everyday life we rarely act with such deliberate intent. Most of the time, we react in habitual ways to situations without thinking too much about what we are doing or whether we might act otherwise. Dr McVie had a style of dealing with stress symptoms and with over-protective parents and he slipped into it without much pondering about choices. Similarly the responses of Angie and her parents to her stomach pains may have been a reflection of their accustomed ways of reacting to one another in the family: the father tense and aggressive, the mother protective and controlling, the daughter sullenly submissive. The more we stress such habitual patterns of response the less we can see relevance in the idea of making choices. The freedom to choose seems crowded out by the

14

force of habit – 'How else would we expect such a daughter/ father/mother/doctor to act?'

Undoubtedly, any hopes for autonomy must be tempered by such realism. People's actions are affected by influences of all kinds, stemming from their personality, social setting and previous experience. According to the philosophical view called determinism, a full understanding of such factors should lead us to reject altogether the notion of free choice. In principle, it is argued, all human behaviour could be fully predicted, if the human sciences were more precise than at present.[9] This view, however, fails to explain adequately the observed capacity of human beings to reflect on their own behaviour and thereby to modify it. We can free ourselves at least partially from force of habit and from external influences by using this capacity to reflect as a self-regulating device. Such reflection can lead us to a conscious and deliberate change in the style of our relationships, to a genuine moral choice. If such choice is not possible, there seems little point in theorizing about morality. Why worry about Angie's future if what is about to happen to her will inevitably take place?

This book proceeds on the assumption that choice is the crux of morality. When patient meets professional, the ability of each to choose will be enhanced if there is more reflection on the factors which influence their actions. First there is the perspective from which each views the situation – the 'facts', as they are seen. Knowledge of the facts shapes choice, yet it is rarely seen how selective this knowledge is. Next there is the character of the helping relationship, moulded by profes-sional training and the expectations of patients, which so influences the manner in which help is offered. Beyond this there is the patient's own world, one often poorly understood in professional health care. This world is in turn affected by the wider society in the form of family, neighbours, social agencies and the boundaries of law. Balanced against all these factors is the ability of all concerned to share responsibility and take reasoned decisions. No truly moral decision can be made unless all this complexity is recognized. In the chapters which follow we shall examine each of these ideas in turn, while continuing to hear the story of Angie and her family.

Exercises

1. Think of a decision you have made recently (not necessarily a professional one). Try to identify factors predisposing you to decide in a particular way. To what extent is it true to say that you were free to choose an alternative line of action? (Individuals' answers to these questions could be used to start a group discussion on freedom and choice.)

2. Often a professional is faced with a question 'Who is my patient?' and a choice must be made between different family members all asking for help in their own way. How might this apply to Dr McVie's visit to the Carters?

3. Explore the problem of choice, autonomy and paternalism raised by the following cases:

Case One: The Choice of Death

A patient with chronic renal failure became more and more unhappy with measures taken to preserve his kidney function and his basic health. One night in a rage he pulled at the 'shunt' in his arm through which he was attached to the kidney machine, and infection resulted. His arm became gangrenous and he refused to allow anyone to operate. He insisted he wanted to die. The renal physician thought he was insane, and called in a psychiatrist. The psychiatrist did not agree, and considered him depressed but sane, and thought he had made a rational choice of death.

(Case collected by the authors)

Case Two: Death of a Schoolboy

David, a schoolboy of 13 years, was the only child of middle-aged parents. One day he was severely injured in the spine as the result of a playground accident at school. When admitted to a paediatric neurosurgical unit it became quickly evident that the damage to the spine was so extensive that David would almost certainly be totally paralysed from the neck down. The boy was fully conscious and obviously very anxious about his condition. After a few hours, his breathing deteriorated rapidly and it became necessary to put him on to a respirator, after performing a tracheostomy under local anaesthetic. At the same time he was given fairly heavy sedation. At this point David's parents approached the consultant and asked whether there was any hope of David avoiding total paralysis. They were told that there was virtually none. They then suggested that no further effort should

16

be made to maintain David's life, because they regarded his condition as one which the boy could never tolerate.

The medical staff were surprised by this request but eventually agreed that David should be taken off antibiotics and given increased sedation. At no point was the boy told what was happening to him or what his true condition was, and when he asked if he was dying this was vehemently denied. After about a day or so he died of respiratory failure.

(Based on a case reported in I.E. Thompson, *Dilemmas of Dying*, Edinburgh University Press, 1979, pp. 127f)

Case Three: Sterilization of a Nineteen Year Old
She was a West Indian girl who had come to Great Britain when she was 12 to live with an aunt following the death of both of her parents in Jamaica. Her father had been a diabetic, her mother a hypertensive who probably died of heart disease. At 14 the patient herself was admitted as an emergency to hospital in hyperglycaemic coma. A diagnosis of diabetes mellitus was sustained, but there were no other physical stigmata of the disease and she was subsequently stabilized on twice daily injections of soluble insulin. At 16 she left home to work as a shop assistant, became pregnant, and miscarried at 12 weeks. A year later she again became pregnant and during this pregnancy the diabetes was not easily controlled and she was admitted twice, once in hyperglycaemic coma and once with hypoglycaemia. The hospital records of the delivery were not available but her baby was born normally at full term weighing 9 lbs. This child was taken into her aunt's family and was being cared for mainly by the aunt, although the patient frequently visited the baby. The patient had recently come on to the general practitioner's list, and had presented with amenorrhoea lasting for three months. On examination she was clearly pregnant and the general practitioner felt that on clinical and social grounds a termination, which she requested, was justified.

A social worker's report revealed that she was living on her own in a single rented room and had had a number of liaisons in the previous three years. The father of her present child seemed unlikely to marry her or set up a stable home. The aunt was unable to cope with any other children and her relationship with the patient had recently been strained. There were no other relatives living in England. The patient had had a number of general practitioners, and appeared never to have had clear contraceptive advice, although she had at one time been told she

17

could never take the pill, and she was unable to tolerate an intrauterine device. She had not used any other form of contraception, nor had her present boyfriend.

The gynaecologist after seeing her wrote to the general practitioner: 'Thank you for referring this patient. I agree to terminate the pregnancy, although at this stage it will have to be by hysterotomy. Incidentally, I have persuaded her to be sterilized.' The latter operation was carried out at the time of the termination.

Three years later, aged 22, the patient was sent again to the gynaecological clinic complaining of dysmenorrhoea. She had severe pain, often making her stay away from work for the three days before her periods, which were heavy. There were no new gynaecological abnormalities. The diabetes was well controlled with glibenclamide, and there was no report of any further diabetic complications. She was well dressed and seemed composed but rather depressed. On discussion it emerged that she now had a steady boyfriend who wished to marry her, but was unlikely to do so until she was pregnant. She was advised that a tubal reanastomosis was most unlikely to restore her fertility.

(From *Journal of Medical Ethics*, vol. i, no. 1 (April 1975), p. 45. A full discussion of this case will be found in the *Journal*, pp. 45–8).

Case Four: Consent by a Psychiatric Patient

A 59-year-old man was referred to a psychiatric hospital because his memory was fading and he felt he was being persecuted. He had been previously well, with no personal or family history of mental illness. He had married at 25, and had had a happy family life. At the time of admission his wife was still working and was living with him, while the two adult children lived nearby. Over the previous few months, however, his personality had begun to change. He had the fixed idea that he was being pursued by the police for some imagined crime, and that his family was planning to kill him. He slept poorly, ate little and 'could not concentrate on anything'. When seen by the psychiatrist he was restless, wearing an anxious expression, and kept wringing his hands and trying to leave the room. He was confused and depressed and was admitted to the ward under the diagnosis of presenile dementia with depression.

On the ward, formal psychological testing showed that his memory was severely impaired while he appeared to have an IQ within the normal range. This suggested diffuse brain damage, as did the EEG. A neurologist noted a large head and extensor plantar responses. The skull radiograph gave a vital clue: it showed an enlarged vault with a small posterior fossa, and suggested to the radiologist hydrocephalus as a result of aqueduct stenosis. He was transferred to a neurosurgical unit, where the diagnosis was confirmed by a lumbar air encephalogram and angiograms. Surgical correction of the hydrocephalus with a ventriculo-atrial shunt was the alternative to long inpatient care with declining mental function. When this was put plainly to the patient, however, he refused any operation on his head. On phenothiazine medication at this point he was less agitated and appeared to have good insight into his situation, in spite of the dementia. For several weeks he was pressed to consider the operation, but he insisted on returning home.

Initially at home he seemed stabilized, but at follow up a deteriorating picture emerged. He became suspicious again and his day-to-day activities diminished. Four months after discharge he became totally disorientated and needed admission under section 29 (72 hours only), which was then converted to section 25 (28 days only). (Both of these sections allow observation but certainly not operative treatment). There was no objective evidence that the dementia had worsened, so although he was confused and initially unable to account for his actions the psychiatrists felt that he had retained insight and was aware that things were not what they had been when he was first admitted. He blamed this deterioration on the doctors: 'They gave me the mind of a baby.' He became more lucid and more understanding on phenothiazines, but continued to deny that he had brain disorder and refused operation. Because of his retained insight the psychiatrists felt that they could not recommend him for operation against his expressed wish, especially as there seemed no clear indication as to how effective and safe the operation might be.

(See *Journal of Medical Ethics*, vol. i, No. 3 (September 1975) for a fuller account of this case and an inter-disciplinary discussion)

2

Facts

The ambulance lay empty at the casualty bay. They had obviously taken the patient inside already. Sheila, the house physician on call, pushed through the rubber doors to the resuscitation bay.

'Oh God, not another one – that's the third arrest tonight.' Sheila's breathlessness was just under control as she relieved the sweating ambulanceman of his job. The charge nurse had already connected the ECG to the arms and was working on the feet. By some miracle, there was a drip running – who could have put that up? Her registrar had just got an airway he was satisfied with, and turned to her with that 'was it the high heels that kept you?' look.

The steady flash of the ambulance's light still forced its way in. It accentuated the blue mottled face, the sightless eyes, the wide black pupils. Sheila's torch flicked across them.

'Are they coming down?'

'Not so far.'

'VF – stand clear' said the registrar quietly. Jelly was smeared: the smell of hot flesh.

'Again – up to 400 please, charge nurse.'

'Ah bingo – sinus: is there an output, Sheila?'

She felt the groin pulse.

'Weak, Geoff, but there – but not every beat.' Her hand felt the characteristic shape of a pill container in the pocket. She glanced at the ambulanceman. 'What do we know about him? Is he an OD?'

'Not likely, Doc, I don't think, though there had been a bit of family dingdong, I gather. He just arrested at home in front of the telly – all smashed it was. Daughter called us – mother was out it seems – very upset. She kept on moaning 'He shouldn't have said it, how could I have known?' but we couldn't find out any more as we had to bring him in. He's bloody young isn't he? – not forty-five yet, daughter said. Makes you think. We got him going pretty quick, I reckon.'

'Remarkable – very well done. He's beating OK now, though not breathing on his own. Mucky job, isn't it – but satisfying. Mucky things can be satisfying, eh Sheila?'

'Oh Geoff, shut up – look at these. Valium. Twenty in there. "A. Carter" – is that him?'

'No, he's John – "A" may be his wife – or the daughter I suppose. Anyway he's stable enough and we can take him down to the ICU. Is that OK, Charge?'

'Yes, fine – but what about the relatives? Can you see them, Sheila?'

'Yes, please do, Sheila. With more details perhaps you'll be able to get a clearer picture of what's going on. Nicotine stains: obviously a heavy smoker. Still, we'll need to know a bit more. I don't want to be gloomy but he was anoxic a long time, and these pupils are still a bit sluggish. Better not say too much to the family yet. Go along and take a history, Sheila, and see what you can find out.'

The house physician left slowly. It was over an hour later when she got to the intensive care unit.

'No neurological response yet', said Sister. 'Looks pretty hopeless doesn't it? What's the matter, Sheila?'

The house physician slumped into a chair. It was the first time she'd cried since she qualified.

Bad Monday afternoons may lead to worse Monday evenings. It was the third arrest that night – just another coronary for the registrar, and satisfying to have got the heart going again. But once that crisis was over, and the resuscitation team had time to catch their breath, another task lay ahead. More information was needed.

The information that the charge nurse needed as Mr Carter was brought in, the details that the registrar noted as he responded to the emergency call, were very straightforward. The ambulanceman added some more and discoveries were made in the resuscitation. But most of this information was geared to the immediate emergency. What Sheila, the house doctor, found out later seemed to be of a different order. What Dr McVie had already discovered was different again. All of them had made estimates of what was going on, had formed initial diagnoses, and reacted accordingly. They noted some things, and ignored others, out of the mass of data available to them. What influenced this selection?

Two Notions

The resuscitation team were interested only in restoring the circulation in a man with a cardiac arrest. To do this, they needed to insert an airway and help him to breathe; they needed to assess the heart's functioning, and keep the heart beating by external massage in the meantime; and they needed to have a drip running, to correct the biochemical 'muddle' caused by circulation failure. To them, and to some readers, this was routine, difficult but not out of the ordinary. To others, even the language is obscure – 'VF', ventricular fibrillation, a chaotic heart rhythm that needs correction by external electrical shock, and 'OD', the possibility that Mr Carter might have taken a drug overdose, which would have created further problems. Each observation led to an action, in a reasonably logical way. To the outsider, a miracle: to the physician, simply the speedy application of certain basic clinical principles. The data were not difficult to gather, and the registrar sent Sheila away to collect more on the structured basis that all learn at Medical School – the history of the present illness, previous problems, allergies and so on. After that, when things had settled down there is general physical examination; while precise measurements of blood pressure, pulse and ECG traces are being carefully checked by the coronary unit staff as part of their job.

Dr McVie's observations were very different from these. Unlike the routine call to the emergency team, he was responding to a request for a visit from a family he already knew. As he went, he ordered this knowledge in his mind. But his response was completely changed by the 'atmosphere' in the house. Was this something he had been taught to observe? How could he have detected it, and how could he measure it? Would he have been able to describe it to anyone? Would the registrar, Geoff, have understood if he had?

The nature of these questions suggests that Geoff and Dr McVie, although trained for the same profession, have learned to collect different types of information in totally different ways. Each set of data is vital to doctor and patient, but difficult to convey to the other if not familiar with the work. Both sets are valid, and give reliable results if used correctly. But each set relates to the *task* of the person gathering it, the aims that he has in 'the management of the case'. This variation can be seen even more clearly if one professional approach is contrasted with another, for example, the approach of a social worker with that of a nurse. So when it is argued that people 'need to know the facts', it first has to be understood that 'the facts' depend on what they have in mind. What is fact and what is not is a judgement. The values that underpin that judgement may be difficult to discern, but they are there of necessity. Facts and values live side by side.

Relevance

Every professional person faces the same difficulty. Each has to develop special skills to gather the 'relevant' data. In the process other skills are neglected. This is necessary in order to reduce the potential chaos of data available. To act differently would be to act less efficiently, and the task might suffer. Thus inevitably professionals must narrow their perspective.

It is hard to connect the Mr Carter seen in the casualty bay with the father first met in the Carters' flat just a few hours earlier. We first saw him through the eyes of a general practitioner, then through those of a hospital emergency team. In a similar way, Angie is at the centre of attention in the Carters' flat, but is reduced to 'a character off-stage' in the hospital. Geoff, Sheila and charge nurse could not have done their job if distracted by Angie, yet Dr McVie's knowledge of Angie is essential if Mr Carter's case is to be understood fully. We might guess that Sheila's tears came through seeing Mr Carter as Angie's dying father. Her perspective had suddenly changed.

What is less often observed is that patients or clients also narrow their perspective with circumstances. A medical problem may be rehearsed with a relative or friend,[1] the decision made to take it to a professional, who may refer to a more specialized worker and so on – at each stage the range of information will get smaller but the data sought on each issue will be greater, or deeper. It is a process not unlike changing the focal length on a camera, or a microscope. At each stage, some things will get clearer – and some things will get completely lost.

We have suggested in the last chapter that the opportunity to make a choice is central to any morally effective encounter, and that choice depends on adequate knowledge of the facts. But now we can see that there are many different styles of gathering relevant information which may be given the status of 'fact'. It is therefore important to look more closely at these different styles since these affect the choices made. This may be illustrated by concentrating on the differences between two medical approaches: the precise measurements of Geoff, medical registrar, and the intuitive insight of Dr McVie.

Science and Rationality

The scientific foundation of the registrar's observations seems very solid. He measures the rate of the pulse, together with the pattern of the electrocardiogram and the circulation produced in the body. Unless he is using faulty techniques or there is a machine error, his observations will be considered entirely reliable. This ability to make measured observations, and to draw conclusions on the basis of which predictions can be made, is central to scientific method. It has revolutionized the practice of modern medicine, to a point where many regard such data as the only relevant and reliable facts.

Is it really so obvious that scientific knowledge rests wholly on solid foundations? Scientific 'facts' tend to be ones which observers readily agree about, as opposed to, say, aesthetic observations which are so much a matter of opinion. What is less often remembered is that there can be no scientific information without an observation and this in itself introduces elements of judgement and uncertainty. There is always the possibility of observer error, and contamination of the observation by what the observer wishes to find: inaccurate blood pressure reading is often quoted as an example of this in clinical practice.

At a more theoretical level, what the future holds cannot be absolutely certain. Thus scientific statements[2] are really

24

predictions relying on probability based on past observation. The observations which underline Mr Carter's poor prognosis fall into this category. Unfortunately where action is demanded undue reliance must be placed on the scanty evidence available, and spurious certainty may be attributed to this by workers in the field to cover their deficiencies.[3] The place of inspired guesswork in pure science sometimes goes unrecognized: in applied science it can hardly be ignored. There is no place for debate on probability theory in the emergency room, any more than there is for a discussion of family dynamics. The problem for medical ethics arises when the style of the emergency room is taken for the norm. This is not to question the importance of scientific observations at any level, but the conclusions that are drawn from such observations, and the use to which they are put, raise different issues. The application of a scientific idea in technology is only as appropriate as the thinking behind it.

Scientific method can be defined too narrowly. Measuring things and applying mathematics to the resulting measurements is often regarded as the corner-stone of scientific thinking. Its success has deceived some into the thought that observation without measurement is not worth doing. It is the method, however, not the means, which is important: the processes of insight, and hypothesis formation, derived from initial observations, followed by the testing or refuting of the hypothesis with further observations, and the logical reasoning that surrounds this testing, are all essential parts of scientific method, with the aim of knowing more, of reducing blurred and incoherent patterns to meaning and coherence.

Intuitive Observation

Turning to Dr McVie, the sceptic might declare that one cannot measure 'atmosphere' in the sense that Dr McVie detected it and that this is a purely subjective judgement which can neither be proved nor refuted. But Dr McVie responded to a sensation inside himself created by a pattern of data perceived at that moment which he recognized as being associated with stress in a small group. The data were different: a way of greeting, tension in the face, closed eyelids, a line of tears, all associated with other details that might not even have been consciously observed. Some would call this simply sensitivity. But the scene and Dr McVie's feelings about it were as much 'signs' as the physical findings in Angie's examination. Having created a hypothesis based on all this, he tested the idea by the means at his disposal in the living laboratory of the flat, and verified the existence of family tension. His methods were thus not so different from Geoff's, but relied on what his body taught him, 'in-tuition', not the external 'hard' data of the cardiac arrest team. The 'soft' data he obtained were valid, and powerful, in view of the task facing him as a family doctor.

The problem that Dr McVie encountered was that he was unable, for many reasons, to enter fully into the 'atmosphere' he had discovered. It seems that Sheila, the house doctor, did go deeper into the situation and, as a result, broke down. We do not know precisely what upset her, but we may guess that round a blind corner she blundered into Angie's grief and guilt, and they bowled her over.

Focus and Perspective

The difficulties that demands of this kind cause may raise moral as well as practical issues. How could Sheila have been helped to cope? Just as we suspect that Dr McVie might not have been very effective at resuscitation, we may suppose that the problems Sheila was faced with were beyond her new, but restricted, clinical skills. Training was suggesting to her that she should not be involved with a patient's non-medical problems, so that she could cope with at least three cardiac arrests in one night. Personal feelings might pull another way: like Angie, she was young and presumably had as deep feelings within herself about fathers as Dr McVie had about children. These feelings gave her insights she had forgotten she had. Clinical observation and personal feelings were perhaps in direct conflict, because they implied a disorientating or even nauseous double perspective on a scene already too sharply in focus for comfort.

Sheila could have taken a history without noticing what was happening within the family. That she did not, and was disturbed by what she learned, is a sign of strength, not weakness – of human success, not clinical failure. Many would not have noticed, and would have diminished themselves and their patients in the process. But she faced the difficulty that may confront anyone who changes viewpoint or focus – they then may see an unfamiliar world. A nurse learns to cope with the stench of a festering wound, but may be totally unable to deal with an angry relative. A social worker, used to helping an individual client, may be lost when trying to deal with a demand that the client be evicted by their own Authority. A surgeon, used to the confusion of bleeding and cancerous bowels, may find that unravelling the muddle of unhappy people is beyond him.

The Response to Uncertainty

It is very interesting to observe what happens when people find themselves in an unknown and potentially threatening landscape. Usually, each person withdraws to familiar ground,[4] or returns to the focus, with which he can cope. The GP prescribes – as he so often does. The registrar goes to ICU – where he feels at home. (Should one add, the philosopher returns quickly to the fence he was sitting on before?) These physical moves symbolize mental shifts: when asked to justify or explain their moves, many professional workers become not more flexible, but more rigid and closed, or in the original analogy, more fixed in their focus.

There are many other pressures that contribute to this. There are the pressures of time. The apparent need to be seen to be making decisions is a habit easily acquired and difficult to relinquish. An anxious patient needs to be re-assured, or a gap in therapy filled – it is easy to be pressed to shift the weight of probabilities and create 'facts' where there are really only vague possibilities. The history of medicine is full of such blind alleys, and many must presumably exist today: but it is more difficult to catch ourselves, as professionals or as patients, playing this game. Studies of the process involved in reaching a diagnosis have shown that the final choice is reached remarkably early in the process – often right at the beginning.[5] First impressions are often right – but

27

incomplete. Both sides of the encounter need information on which to base their decisions. Which 'facts' are chosen to transmit to the other side is crucial to the outcome. Does the cardiologist need or want to know about my recent affair at the office? Should he tell me that the slightly ischaemic pattern on the ECG is normal for my age or that it is an indication of heart disease?

Trying to apply scientific thinking to everyday work may be an uncomfortable process. There are difficulties in the boundaries between research and treatment – in the application of statistical data to the individual patient for instance: and in the boundaries between the measurable and controllable and the immeasurable and unexpected – for example, the role of medicine in the natural processes of birth and death. Part of this may result from our restricted and inflexible understanding of scientific probability. There are enormous limitations still to scientific knowledge, and in addition no one can have access to all that is available. Thus, professionals feel uncertain because they realize they have incomplete mastery of available knowledge. But the normal uncertainties of clinical practice go beyond this. They lie in the difficulty in focusing on what are the relevant areas to study in the individual case, and in being able to change that focus and retain our power to help. Sheila can be helped by learning more about the uncertainties of her work, and about how to tolerate and use those uncertainties as one of the major strengths of clinical or social work.

Facts and Moral Choice

We began by acknowledging that there were no absolute facts, only facts seen from a specific perspective. We examined two, amongst many such perspectives, and concluded that the professional must be flexible enough to change focus when this is required. The feelings of uncertainty that this arouses need to be coped with positively. That many people either do not change focus, or cannot cope with the consequences, is a practical and moral issue: and the practical failures in their turn produce moral problems.

This interrelationship between shifting perspective and

28

moral choice is evident in the second episode of Angie's story. The decisions to be taken by the cardiac arrest team were in a sense routine. Later in Mr Carter's treatment, were he to survive without further recovery, more difficult choices might arise. But still in the immediate situation there was the less obvious issue of the effects of his collapse on the Carter family. This emerged when Sheila shifted her perspective on the facts.

Just as Dr McVie's response to Angie in the flat might have altered the outcome, so now the response of the medical and nursing team in the hospital might well modify the future for this family. Once again the practical and the moral intertwine. Can anything be done to help the family now, and if so, who will help Angie and her mother in the crisis that now engulfs them? Is this the responsibility of the hospital at all? Was Sheila too sensitive and were her tears inappropriate? She now had access to a whole range of new information which opened fresh choices for her as a doctor, yet is it her business to get involved? If it is not, whose business is it? This raises the whole question of the role and response of the professional, which will be the subject of the next chapter.

Exercises

1. Consider the *focus* and *perspective* of the case histories, reports or assessments which you prepare in your professional work. What assumptions about relevance are made in such standardized records? Which aspects of the patient's or client's experience might be overlooked by them? (If you are not a professional worker, try to recall a visit to a doctor or other professional. What 'facts' did you come prepared with, prior to the interview? Pay particular attention to information you discounted as irrelevant.)

2. In the *Doctor-Patient Relationship* by K. Browne and P. Freeling (Churchill Livingstone, 1976, ch. 7) doctors are advised to observe the effects patients are having on them, as an aid to understanding their patients better. Try to recall an incident in your experience of helping people which demonstrates the usefulness of this approach. (Answers may be used to start a group discussion.)

3. Have people the right to demand that information held in their medical records should be deleted? Consider this question in relation to the following case, or other cases in your experience.

Mr and Mrs Spence

Mrs Spence had considerable trouble in obtaining her present pregnancy. She was the wife of a teacher who was about to leave the locality to take up the post of a headmaster at a boys' public school. Mrs Spence had also been a teacher, but was now not working as she was pregnant. During her previous marriage she had been pregnant and miscarried twice; in fact had never carried a baby to full term. Her previous husband had left her and she felt that her miscarriages had partly contributed to the breakdown of their relationship. Her present marriage was five years old. It had rapidly become clear that they needed infertility investigations and were referred to a private clinic. Here her present husband was found to be infertile and they requested and were accepted for artificial insemination by donor. Because of her previous miscarriages Mrs Spence had a series of hormone injections given by her general practitioner in the early months of her pregnancy. At the last of these consultations, when she was about to leave the practice because of their move to the new district, Mrs Spence asked her doctor to destroy any record of the artificial insemination so that no one would know about it. She said that she and her husband had discussed this at length, and that they wanted to make a new start, and felt it would be fairer on the child if nothing were known about this. Her general practitioner reluctantly agreed.

(See *Journal of Medical Ethics*, 1978, no. 4, 207–9 for a discussion of this case)

4. The following extract from *The Psychology of Consciousness* by Robert E. Ornstein (Harcourt, Brace & Jovanovich, New York 1977) argues that (a) personal consciousness is a radically selective picture of 'reality' (b) the consciousness we construct is primarily determined by the need to survive. Consider the relevance of these ideas to the respective viewpoints of patients and professionals.

Even a moment's reflection will confirm that our general idea of a personal consciousness as a perfect mirror of an external reality cannot be true. . .

Consider . . . the enormous variety of physical energies that we contact at each moment of our lives. The air, or more properly, the atmospheric environment, conveys energy in the electromagnetic band: visible light, X-rays, radio waves, infra-red radiation. In addition, there is present the mechanical vibration of the air, containing the information of sound; the constant energy from the gravitational field; pressure on the body; gaseous matter in the air. We also generate our own internal stimuli – thoughts, internal organ sensations, muscular activity, pains, feelings, and much more. These processes are always occurring simultaneously and continue as long as we are alive; yet we are certainly not aware of *each* process at *each* moment. Our personal consciousness, then, cannot fully represent the external world or even our internal world but must consist of an extremely small fraction of the entire 'reality'. We do not even possess the sensory systems to perceive many forms of available energy, such as ultraviolet radiation.

Many questions arise once we realize that our personal consciousness is extremely limited. How do we manage to maintain a relatively stable personal consciousness in the face of all the stimuli that impinge on us? What is the nature of our experience of the world? Why is it necessary for our personal consciousness to be so limited?

Personal consciousness is outward oriented, involving action, for the most part. It is most likely to have evolved for the primary purpose of ensuring individual biological survival, for which active manipulation of discrete objects, sensitivity to threatening organisms or forces that pose a threat, and separation of oneself

31

from others would have been useful. Our biological inheritance determines that we *select* the sensory personal consciousness from the mass of information reaching us. This is done by a multilevel process of filtration, for the most part sorting out survival-related stimuli. From this, we are ultimately able to *construct* a stable consciousness in co-ordination with the filtered input.

(*The Psychology of Consciousness*,
pp.42f)

3

Cases

Sister Curran stopped her cortège of new nurses by the first incubator.

'Let's start by looking a little closer at this case, shall we, since it's the first time most of you have actually been on the neonatal unit here. This is baby Carter, and he is an important example of what can be done in a special care baby unit. What do you notice about him?'

Five pairs of eyes peered anxiously at the tiny form, and five identical pairs of eyes stared back at them from the glass, as if defying them to find the words they wanted.

'He's very skinny, Sister – and his feet are so tiny compared with his head.'

'Yes, Baby Carter was born at 35 weeks gestation, and so is a "preterm" baby. But as you can see, two weeks later he is still in an incubator, we are still having to tube feed him, and he is still below this line here on the chart which indicates the weight we would like him to be. So he is also "light for dates" – do you know why that is?'

'I suppose because he wasn't nourished enough in the womb.'

'Yes nurse.' Sister surveyed the plump figure who had spoken. 'It is important to get nutrition right. Baby Carter started out all right at the beginning of the pregnancy, and his brain grew satisfactorily, but something seems to have gone wrong later, hence the skinny legs. He'll catch up eventually, but while he is so vulnerable it is very important to keep up the blood sugar with regular feeds, keep him warm, and prevent any cross-infection by being scrupulous with handwashing – like that nurse over there is doing.'

'What went wrong with Baby Carter, Sister?'

'Well, yes, a very interesting and distressing case. His mother is sixteen and not married. I'm not sure what's become of the baby's father, but the young girl, Angie Carter, seems to have concealed the pregnancy till quite late on, and then perhaps tried to hide her condition by starving. So she booked late, and was smoking too – both pointers to an "at risk" pregnancy.'

'Is that why he was born prematurely?'

'Labour started when the mother took an overdose, and the baby was born in rather unfortunate circumstances in casualty with a low Apgar score. Do you know what that is?'

'Isn't it a measure of the baby's responses, Sister, when he is first born?'

'Good. Baby Carter scored 6,7,7. What does that suggest?'

The group looked in silence from the numbers to the distant little figure, naked except for a pair of huge white gloves and a plastic bag for urine. It seemed a wonder that this scrap had scored anything at all.

'Well, it indicates that the baby was not very responsive at the beginning and didn't improve very much subsequently – probably a result of mother's overdose.'

'What's happened to her, Sister – is she on the ward here now?'

'No, unfortunately. She had a severe post-partum haemorrhage. After she had got over that she was at first very withdrawn and then she began to behave in a rather disturbed way, and got very aggressive. Apparently her father had died suddenly at the beginning of the pregnancy and she had reacted very badly to that. We were about to have her seen by the psychiatrists, but she discharged herself and we didn't feel we were able to try to keep her in. Now she comes up every day with the grandmother. I'm pressing her to come in again, but she doesn't seem to know her own mind at the moment.'

'What's the outlook, Sister, do you think?'

'The prognosis? For Baby Carter, fairly reasonable I should say, although he's by no means out of the wood yet. But for the family, or rather the mother, I'd hate to predict. She certainly is a case.'

So, Angie is a case. Since we last heard about her, her father has died, she has gone through a pregnancy and delivered prematurely. It was a very disturbing time – she became depressed in trying to conceal the pregnancy, treated herself unwisely, and took an overdose. The delivery was nearly a disaster and she bled badly. So many mishaps in such a short time must be enough to make anyone a hospital case. And Sister Curran feels just that.

But what would Sister Curran and her nurses do without her or someone like her? It takes two to make a case. Patients or clients are as necessary to nurses, doctors or social workers as machines to mechanics. Whether the work is seen as a job, vocation, role or the curse of the drinking classes, few professionals can avoid it dominating their thoughts and attitudes for much of the day. Even hanging up the white coat, leaving the files behind or taking a holiday can be difficult.

In a similar way, people can become dedicated to the career of being a patient. Every hospital or practice has its share of 'regulars' whose illnesses may come and go, but whose status as a patient keeps them in permanent touch with the health services. To remain somebody's case becomes part of their identity. Perhaps this is beginning to happen to Angie.

If anyone can be a patient, not everyone need be a case. Sister Curran thought Angie was a case almost in the colloquial sense, like 'oh you are a one'. Sometimes it is used by patients themselves in more precise terms. 'Am I a case?', said an old lady to her doctor, as she recounted the terrors of an evening when she was sure she had heard her recently dead husband's key in the lock and smelt his pipe, at the time when he used to come home from work. To be reassured and comforted, she not only needed to be told that this was part of a normal bereavement reaction, but that she was not mentally unbalanced, about to 'go mad'. By appearing in the surgery, she announced herself as a patient: to become a case was a much more serious step.

In order to study the moral consequences of the interdependence of patient and professional involved in 'being a case', it is necessary to look more carefully at the style of encounter that may be adopted. One way to observe this is to consider what happens to people in professional training. How do they learn to act in a professional manner? What responses do they learn to expect from patients or clients?

Professional Detachment

The need for some sort of stance in professional relationships different from that of a friend or neighbour becomes obvious as soon as the raw student enters a ward round or an office.

The complexity of information which was discussed in the last chapter can become random and unintelligible 'white noise' to the newcomer who is desperately trying to make sense of what she or he hears, and link it to some of the concepts that have been taught, in the ward or classroom.

Every gain involves some loss. The student gains control, while losing many facets that patients would like her or him to retain. Inevitably, there is a distancing process; it is impossible to become involved with so many problems. The sensitivity that most of us have to other people's needs and attitudes is made subservient to the two tasks in hand, to gain information and to learn how to deal with the patient's illness. That neither of these necessarily always benefits that patient is an unpleasant thought that is tucked away quickly. It takes an unusual comment to alert us to the enormous shift in attitudes that most nursing, medical or social work students have to undergo. Students sometimes draw attention to this:

'I feel quite superfluous, an intruder. We have no right to ask these questions.' 'Why does a doctor always use such a funny voice?'[1]

A medical student, contemplating her final exams, declared to a clinical teacher: 'I am no longer sure that I want to be a doctor. I don't want to become like you.'[2]

It must be impossible to manipulate (often in unpleasant circumstances) the human body of a stranger, with all its attendant taboos, without acquiring new attitudes. Indeed learning anatomy on a cadaver may be more useful as a 'deep-end' introduction to this aspect of professional work than the knowledge of the body that is gained. Likewise nurses who learn the techniques of laying out the corpse are being taught an emotional attitude as much as a technical nursing skill. George Orwell writes of his examination by students in a Paris Hospital:

> . . . if you had some disease with which the students wanted to familiarize themselves you got plenty of attention of a kind. I myself, with an exceptionally fine specimen of bronchial rattle, sometimes had as many as a dozen students queueing up to listen to my chest. It was a queer feeling – queer, I mean, because of their intense interest in learning

their job, together with a seeming lack of any perception that the patients were human beings. It is strange to relate, but sometimes as some young student stepped forward to take his turn at manipulating you he would be actually tremulous with excitement, like a boy who has at last got his hands on some expensive piece of machinery. And then ear after ear – ears of young men, of girls, of Negroes – pressed against your back, relays of fingers solemnly but clumsily tapping, and not from any one of them did you get a word of conversation or a look – direct in your face. As a non-paying patient in the uniform nightshirt, you were primarily *a specimen*, a thing I did not resent, but could never quite get used to.[3]

All professional workers do at times need to be objective and detached, and will damage their clients if they are not. As 'the greatest art is to know when to apply the science', so the greatest skill may be to be able to think logically and objectively for a client while responding to him in a warm and empathic way. That few achieve it fully in a medical context may be a cause for concern, but perhaps not for complaint. In the more rigorously scientific conditions of clinical research, *not* to act in a detached 'double blind' way[4] might be unethical since it would allow subjective bias to influence the assessment of the effectiveness of treatment. But the worker involved in an experiment who does not distinguish between the needs of science and the needs of his patient can be on very dangerous moral ground.[5]

Vocation and Consistency

A second feature of learning to act professionally is the acquisition of an impartial and consistent approach to patients. This manifests itself in the professional 'manner' of doctor, nurse, social worker or clergyman, which is often caricatured in literature or the theatre. A classic description of the traditional medical 'manner' is given in the Code of Ethics of the American Medical Association of 1847:

Physicians should study also their deportment so as to unite tenderness with firmness, and condescension with authority, so as to inspire the minds of their patients with gratitude, respect and confidence.

Few people would want to emulate this approach today, but we must not overlook the importance for the patient of some predictable and consistent style of professional behaviour. The professional helper who just wants to be 'a person like anyone else' lays himself or herself open to all kinds of subjective bias. Consistent impartiality may not come easily to those who have not sorted out their own attitudes, or have sorted them out all too well. For example, clinical judgements about a patient who arouses strong antipathetic feelings may be hard to make. As we hear on Sister Curran's teaching round the description of Angie's more recent behaviour, we begin to sense elements that might alienate her from the sympathy of less perceptive staff.

Unfortunately, professional training cannot eliminate all bias and prejudice. Indeed it may in some respects increase them by underlining the attitudes and values of the 'professional classes'. Many studies have shown that health care workers spend more time with the type of patient they like or understand – for example, with their middle-class patients.[6] When matched with the reported increased incidence of pathology in the lower socio-economic groups, this understandable but inequitable behaviour reveals itself as another example of the 'inverse care law'.[7] The balance between a consistent professional approach, irrespective of personal feelings, and an openness towards the uniqueness and special circumstances of each patient is not easy to maintain. Yet it is this balance which is the essence of genuine help.

Curing and Caring

A third feature of professional training is an unresolved tension between cure and care in modern medicine. Angie and her baby are both cases, but as far as the maternity ward is concerned once Angie's haemorrhage has been dealt with her problems seem singularly intractable. The baby has identifiable physical problems which are difficult but well within the capacity of the ward to solve. But Angie rapidly ceases to be a 'suitable case for treatment'. She is a 'difficult patient' whose behaviour puts her beyond the reach of the staff. Eventually she resolves their dilemma by discharging herself.

There is nothing particularly surprising about this response to Angie. Sadly, things often turn out this way. Most doctors show a preference for dealing with patients whose problems are acute, physical and curable.[8] Everyone likes to get results, yet how commonly do we actually get them? Most modern health problems are chronic and incurable, yet the preference continues. This perhaps derives from the hierarchies of status within medicine (for example, the neurosurgeon is more highly regarded than the geriatrician) and from the excitement of the 'detective game'. Within this system the rarest diagnosis is one of 'health'. Few patients are ever allowed to leave a hospital without a condition of some sort being diagnosed (even if it is only iron deficiency anaemia after multiple blood tests, as one cynic once remarked!). In the law, every person is innocent until proved guilty: within a medical environment, everyone is ill until proved well.[9] If no physical illness is eventually found, the person runs the risk of being rejected as a 'failed patient'.

This preference for identifying disease and achieving cures affects the other professions involved in health care. 'Professions ancillary to medicine' may be required to act as if only in a handmaiden role to the curative ministrations of doctors instead of developing their own skills. Social work is often regarded as suspect because it has no obviously curative effect. General nurses may try to bask in the reflected glory of acute medicine, seeing speedy physical recovery as their prime aim. These attitudes totally ignore the real situation in which dramatic cures are the exception, and a large part of professional work is educative and supportive, mobilizing the patient's resources to meet the irremediable features of an illness or disability.

Anonymity and Organization

A final feature of professional training is learning to work with others as part of an organization. The organization of health care may appear to create further distance between the patient and the source of decisions about his or her care, with patient and practitioner becoming cogs in a bureaucratic machine. This is as true of private medical care as of services organized by the state. Even the traditional single-handed practitioner, who might appear to be very much a free agent dealing directly with individuals, cannot avoid offering his services within a system which has its defined categories of illness and its routines and regulations for treatment. For some purposes the individual features of professionals and patients must be largely ignored in the interests of devising units of measurement – for bed numbers, staffing ratios, average case loads, and so on. Patients must become anonymous to be counted in the statistics which ensure that their care is effectively planned. The practitioner must act within the system, providing services in a way which is allowed for by the design of the system as a whole. One cog must mesh properly with another in order for the machine to keep turning.

But here the analogy must cease. It is the job of professionals to use and interpret the system for the patient's benefit. To act without thought for the individual's needs is to alienate the patient from the system and the worker from his task.

A specific example of how professionals may allow themselves to be seduced by the system within which they work has been called the 'collusion of anonymity'.[10] Here the patient becomes lost between referring specialists or agencies who hand him or her back and forth, with no one taking ultimate responsibility – a case, but no one's case in particular. Were Angie's needs missed at this point because they were not seen, or because her problems were passed between nurses, obstetricians, psychiatrists and social workers? No one particular person seems to have shown Angie that he or she could take her case in hand, could mobilize the help she needed, and set things moving in the right way for her. Feeling lost amongst strangers, she left.

Anonymity is a game professionals often play. In an emergency a person does not object to being seen merely as a post-partum haemorrhage and to being treated by someone who concentrates solely on being an efficient pair of surgical hands. This use of anonymity is transitory – and it will prob-

ably help to save life. The trouble arises when the game is
played with such persistence that it can never be abandoned.
The patient becomes labelled with a disease in a way that
closes off any understanding of him or her as an individual.
Angie is an 'OD', a 'depressive', or a 'suicide risk'. The labels
stick. But while some labels are dangerous others may be
lethal. These may prevent individuals from receiving further
help, and limit the liability of the system:

> A 34-year-old office worker developed psychotic symptoms
> and went 'on the drift'. He drank heavily and had a serious
> road accident which caused brain damage and epilepsy. As
> an alcoholic and epileptic, lodging houses would not accept
> him for long, and no psychiatric hospital would take re-
> sponsibility for him. He died while sleeping rough in South
> London.[11]

The Case and the Whole Person

The features of the professional role which we have now
surveyed – detachment, consistency, the tension between cure
and care and working within an organization – all have a
positive part to play. The sentimentalist who supposes that
'tender loving care' is all that is needed to make a good
doctor, nurse or social worker must soon be disabused of this
illusion. A professional must be able to offer help to seemingly
unlovable people too. However, close almost loving relationships can have a damaging effect if all they do is create
dependency. Seeing patients mainly as 'cases' is a way of
protecting them from being taken over or smothered by
over-involved helpers. It leaves people free to accept the limited help which the professional can offer, and then to detach
themselves from the relationship when its purpose has been
achieved and get on with living their own lives.

A professional relationship is neither a wholly personal nor
wholly impersonal relationship. A patient or client is different
from a friend or relative: but also different from an object
which may be examined and manipulated at will. It has
become fashionable to talk of 'whole person medicine', by
which is meant that physical, psychological and social factors

41

must all be taken into account when seeking to understand a person's illness. This concept is related to the definition of health adopted by the World Health Organization in its Charter:

> Health is a state of complete physical, mental and social well-being and not merely the absence of disease or infirmity.

This definition has been criticized for being unrealistic, the statement of an unattainable ideal.[12] No doubt this is true. Time alone prevents professional workers from dealing so comprehensively with their patients' lives and a person so comprehensively healthy is hard to find. Moreover, the attempt to practise 'whole person medicine' could give health professions an elevated idea of their own importance, making them into the architects of other people's happiness, when really they are relatively marginal influences in people's lives. But, provided we remember that the WHO definition is providing a goal *for the patient*, it can provide a corrective to a too narrow and impersonal approach to people in professional work. If professional interventions inhibit the development of individuals towards this comprehensive state of well-being then they have lost sight of the whole person in an enthusiasm for dealing efficiently with their case.

Angie, 'the case', provides a full illustration of the issues with which this chapter has been concerned. The nurses on the ward round were learning how to take a professional view of baby Carter and his mother. To do this they had to understand not just the physical aspects of the birth and the baby's subsequent development, but also the psychological and social factors affecting the relationship between mother and child. All this entailed a relatively detached view of the situation, seeing both Angie and her baby as examples of mothers and babies of a particular kind. The baby could be seen as an 'at risk' baby. Angie is a potentially 'incompetent mum' who would need to be helped to cope properly. The distance gives the professional staff perspective on the problems. A case-centred approach prevents the emotional over-involvement which might have been natural for a group of young women who themselves could be mothers one day.

Yet this same approach leaves the nursing staff wholly in the dark about Angie, and unable to help her. Sooner or later her baby will be going home and all the hospital can hope for is that someone in the community services will take on the responsibility of seeing that he is cared for adequately. Angie has become 'a case' in the bad sense for the hospital staff – a difficult patient, someone they can't cope with, someone who doesn't fit their system of care. Perhaps the saddest thing is that the professional approach prevents the hospital staff from seeing the seriousness of their failure. The language they use allows them to describe everything as *Angie's* inadequacy, not their own or the system's. None of the nurses asks why a very young unmarried girl having her first baby after a recent bereavement was left feeling helpless and inadequate, alienated from the paediatric ward and from her child. The atmosphere of the ward round does not encourage questions like this. Yet from the point of view of Angie's future life with her baby, this sad and confusing beginning is as serious a threat to health as all the physical aspects so carefully monitored and controlled by the hospital. It seems that Angie is one step further along the road that leads to illness as a way of life, of being a 'case' who fills up the record cards of numerous professional agencies, yet somehow eludes them all. Will someone be willing to break out of the professional mould for the moment and struggle to see Angie through her own eyes? – to ask the seeming unanswerable question, what does it mean to Angie to be Angie?

Exercises

1. Re-read the episode of 'Angie' at the beginning of this chapter. Assess (from your professional or personal perspective) the way in which the situation following the birth of the baby was handled. What might have been done to improve the situation?

2. The following description comes from the diary of a British patient who watched from close quarters a teaching round on a fellow patient from Nigeria. Identify the aspects of the doctor's and students' behaviour which led to the patients' feelings of outrage. How could these have been prevented?

About 4.00 p.m. the door was thrown wide open, and about sixteen men and three or four women, with some overseas students among them, erupted into the room with a teaching doctor. All were listening to the teacher still in full flood of lecturing about the cases just seen. No one looked, nodded, smiled or greeted us in any way. After a few minutes standing in the middle of the room surrounded by his attentive class, he walked over to Mrs A's bed, and after greeting her, began without further preliminaries to 'teach on' her. A student was invited to make an examination; he did not do it very well, stumbling and hesitating, and eventually causing the whole group to laugh. . . The group discussed Mrs A in an impersonal fashion, emphasized. . . by the lecturer's habit of addressing her as Madam. . . Several students were invited to palpate her, and there was considerable to and fro talk over her head throughout the lesson, which lasted about thirty-five minutes. Somewhere in the middle of all this, it occurred to one student to go over and shut the door, which had been left wide open all this time.

. . .there was talk of the difficulty of recognizing yellowness in the whites of the eyes 'in these people', and something about the bodily structure of 'negroid races'. . .No curtains were drawn, but the student crowd hid her from us, although I understand that she was uncovered throughout the session. After it was over, the lecturer left the ward without a word to anyone, nor did most of the students look at the rest of us. In fact, they noticeably guarded themselves from looking at us. Mrs A. was really very incensed, and loudly insisted that such exposure would have been impossible in Nigeria. Sister popped her head in to announce supper which put a stop to the indignation meeting we were all having.

(From G. Horobin, *Medical Encounters*, Croom Helm 1977, pp. 154 f)

3. Case notes are usually not seen by patients or clients. The following incident (described in *The Journal of Medical Ethics*) illustrates what can happen when such notes are seen accidentally. Discuss arguments for and against giving people access to their own case records.

Maria

Maria presented herself in tears to her local advice bureau complaining that her doctor was not only not helping her but had also written insulting remarks about her in her notes. She was a 22-year-old who worked for a London fashion firm: her parents were from Cyprus, but she had been born and brought up in England. She had been to her general practitioner a number of times, she stated, during the previous three months complaining of headaches, which started when at work and lasted well into the evening. She found herself increasingly unable to do her job which she felt she was well suited to and usually enjoyed. As part of the investigation into these headaches she had been referred to her local hospital for tests, which had included X-rays of her skull and a blood test. The blood test raised the possibility that she was suffering from Thalassaemia Minor, and the pathologist asked her to be sent for further tests. After hearing this news, Maria left her doctor's surgery in panic, as she knew one of her mother's sisters had been suffering from this condition and had died in her teens in unpleasant circumstances in Cyprus. Maria presented herself in the Casualty Department of her local hospital that evening with hyperventilation tetany and was later discharged, remembering little of what had gone on, with an appointment to see a psychiatrist at the hospital three weeks later. She could not remember anyone making any further explanations to her. She then returned to her general practitioner. Her doctor worked upstairs in his practice, and patients about to see him would sit upstairs outside his door with their notes. So anxious was Maria that she took out her notes and read them while waiting, 'in order to get to the bottom of the whole thing'. She was appalled to find that the doctor had written at the heading of the page 'Beware, hysterical and manipulative, determined to be unwell.' She had left the surgery at once to seek advice from the bureau.

(See *Journal of Medical Ethics*, 1978, no. 4, pp.207–9 for a discussion of this incident.)

45

4. How far does professional responsibility extend? What responsibility has the psychiatrist got for the suicide in the following case?

Sybil was a 27-year-old single girl who had a good science degree from an English university and had been working in a research post for two years before her first contact with psychiatrists following an overdose. It was noted that this incident was closely related in time to her being offered a position of greater responsibility.

On admission she was thought to have a depressive illness and was treated by a colleague with anti-depressant drugs, and, some weeks later when she showed no response to these, with ECT. She did not change significantly and twice tried to kill herself while in the ward. After four months she was transferred to my care as it was felt she needed more nursing supervision at night which was not available in the first ward. She remained morose, gloomy and continually confronted those around her with her wish to die. In other respects she was intelligent, quite active and did not show any classical features of depressive psychosis.

She was an only child of academic parents and had lived a rather solitary life at home, even when attending university. Although she had few friends she seemed over the years to be making a superficially adequate adjustment to life because of her prowess in passing exams. She had had polio as a child and one leg was somewhat deformed. She felt that this rendered her unattractive, particularly to men. She had had no sexual experience.

Her stay in hospital was turbulent and prolonged. She would engage nurses in long discussions about the purpose of life and present her own case for wishing to end it. Many of the nurses who were closest to her found this experience very distressing and regular team discussions usually divided between those who regarded her wish to die as an illness and those who felt it to be the outcome of her particular view of life but not evidence of pathology. This debate was also reflected in those who wished to restrict her freedom by compulsion if necessary and those who believed this to be unjustified. Initially she was under constant observation and made several further serious attempts on her life; although her attitude remained unchanged, the attempts became less frequent and she was given greater independence. She left to live in a hostel after 18 months and attended twice weekly for outpatient psychotherapy. She continued to say she would kill herself but seemed to be coping. She did successfully commit suicide after an outpatient session and was found dead in a friend's flat.

Two months later I received the first of a series of critical letters from Sybil's mother implying that I had 'let this sick girl die'.

(See *Journal of Medical Ethics*, 1977, no. 3, pp. 93–7 for a discussion of this case.)

5. Consider the following problem from the point of view of each of the three persons mentioned. What rules for procedure could be advanced which would have avoided this outcome? Groups might wish to role play discussion within the surgical team before and after the incident (given a range of attitudes amongst the staff) and the next meeting between patient, relative and staff.

A doctor visited his mother recovering from a gall bladder operation in a teaching hospital, and was alarmed to notice that she was beginning to be jaundiced. When he managed to check this with the House Surgeon, he was told 'Thank you, I'll check this out – it may be to do with the liver biopsy she had.' When the son, astounded, asked further questions the embarrassed houseman admitted that this was a standard procedure in their team and was part of a research project. No permission for this had been sought or obtained before the operation.

(Case collected by the authors)

4

Persons

Mrs Jarvis clashed the gears as she drove away. In all her years as a mother and health visitor, she had never really got used to the smell of baby's vomit. It seemed to linger in the car with her. It had certainly taken over the flat. An odd thing, smell. It's the meaning that deceives the mind. Delicious French cheese, or smelly feet – the paradox of the senses. But all that vomit was a clear message this time. Assuming the doctor was right and there was no pyloric stenosis, there seemed to be a feeding problem, and she must spend more time there. What a tragic story – it's not surprising that this girl couldn't get herself together to be a proper mother, and at sixteen too.

Red lights: she nearly went through.

There had been a bit of an awkward silence when she'd first arrived. She'd heard so much about Angie at the Health Centre that she expected a difficult interview and was surprised in a way that it wasn't a hostile one. Something was odd, apart from the feeding. The baby had seemed all right, sleeping soundly under a bright yellow blanket. It was Angie that took her attention.

The car behind honked. The lights had changed and Angie's words came back to her as if she were still hearing them.

'I never ever thought it would turn out like this. Look how it is – the fire and the frying pan, the pot and the kettle – all black. And me, when will it be me? He's gone and he's come; and he'll never come again, however much I lie on my back and groan here. He's out there, looking in, and *he's* in here, looking out.'

Mrs Jarvis hadn't understood it all, but maybe she would soon.

Angie had begun to tremble – perhaps it was the cold, Mrs Jarvis had hoped, feeling a prickling at the back of her scalp.

'I know you've had a rough time – and are still having it. How is baby?'

Angie had jumped as if she'd forgotten anyone else was there, and had just been reminded. Suddenly words began to flow.

'Yes I know I've got him' – at last she nodded towards the bundle in the cradle – 'and it's wonderful and all that. Mum keeps reminding me – "Be positive" she says – funny thing isn't it, that's my blood group. All those bottles, just to keep me alive. Terribly rare, very important. They told me I'd bled and bled after I had him, though I can't remember much about it. It all blurs together, those times in the Casualty. Always pain, and I can't remember which bit was me, and which bit was . . .'

Her voice had trailed off, she was returning to her dream. 'What happened after he was born?' Mrs Jarvis pulled her back.

'When? Oh, then. Of course, he was taken away – well they said it wasn't like that, but it was, wasn't it? He was in a glass box, for the sake of his life, and it was all touch and go. Yes, it was the best thing for him. But what about me? It was certainly touch and go all right – just open the portholes, touch him and go. No holding him, no bathing him, just touching those tiny little claws and then go. I ached to get hold of him – he was mine after all, wasn't he? – but they wouldn't let me. I was all ache. I think they thought I was too balmy, or stupid or something. I might drop him, or hold him upside down or give him tea instead of milk – some silly ideas anyway, and other mothers with kids just as small were being allowed to hold theirs – so why not me? Why not – when will it ever be my turn?'

'I know I was fuddled then – but I see clearly now, horribly clearly. I was fuddled, and they were a bit frightened. I could tell. They're not used to people being dotty, and "after all you've been through dear". All I've been through indeed – I've never been through anything. I'm always stuck halfway, half in, half out.'

She laughed rather wildly at it all.

'They were so alarmed at what I used to do, they used to walk past as if I had bloody double yellow lines round me and they'd get a parking ticket from Matron or God Almighty if they put their arses on my contaminated bed. I sent one packing – the woman doctor who saw me the night he – my dad – died, and asked lots of questions. 'I know how you feel' she said – though I suppose now she meant it. She came quite a lot, as she'd been there when he'd been born too, she said. But I didn't realize and started to scream at her. How could she know how I felt? No one could know how I felt. Always 'do this', 'do that' at home. I must get on with homework. The only kind words were from Dad, and now he's gone. Mum treats me like an article for display in the window – or did, till I got shop soiled, chipped, marked down. She never cuddled *me*,

now she wants to cuddle *him* all the time. But he's all I've got –
can't she see? Can't she feel how I feel? She suffocates me, I can't
stand it – so that's why I wanted out, a place of my own, on my
own, and that's what I've got now haven't I? I'm on my own, just
me and Jason. Alone with him, and cold like the fridge, inside and
out. I worry about him, you know.'

They had gone over to look at the bundle in the yellow blanket.
Jason and his golden fleece, smiled Mrs Jarvis, remembering school-
days long ago. There was a long voyage ahead for him.

It was Angie who took Mrs Jarvis's attention. The reader
may share with the health visitor the mixed anxiety and relief
that, having seen Angie through so many other people's eyes,
she was now meeting her face to face and hearing how she
was really thinking. It is surprising how rarely people meet
like this. Much contact between people is ritualized, the more
so when clear roles are assumed, as in the medical encounter,
to cope with the stresses, uncertainties and confusions. Professions may alter the mode of perception, increase the distance
between the actors, and reduce, subtly but definitely, the
patients' range of choice. Sometimes this will be a necessity:
sometimes a relief. But sometimes, it seems a denial of all
that health stands for. Angie expresses her criticism – 'When
will it be me?'

It is a challenge of some importance that so little since
Angie's teenage crisis (some might even add since her birth),
seems to have been truly in her hands. Guided and controlled
by caring and careful parents, who wished to steer her safely
through what they saw as a hostile environment, she responded dutifully and intelligently. In their family, the usual
parental behaviours were reversed – but no matter, since
there was both warmth and guidance. But she was growing
up, and the forces of development created, as they must do
in most of us, the desperate need to establish her separate
individual worth and identity, in her own eyes and that of
the community. 'When will it be me?'

These forces created a vacuum, and into this vacuum came
sexual passion. Here was, at last, a chance to achieve all her
body ached for, an understanding of herself, as free. In some

cultures this process of becoming adult is ritualized by a rite of passage, a ceremony, not a wild destructive urge that passed like a seismic shock wave through the whole family and left them isolated and damaged. We have heard little of Tony, the boyfriend, but if the parents were right his elusiveness outlines the ruins of Angie's hopes with even greater clarity. Thomas Hardy, musing on Tess of the D'Urbervilles in similar circumstances, wonders 'Why so often the coarse appropriates the finer thus, the wrong man the woman, the wrong woman the man, many thousands of years of analytical philosophy have failed to explain to our sense of order.'[1]

If Angie was helpless and unprepared in the face of overwhelming and conflicting emotions, so now she appears totally isolated, behind the double yellow lines, in the contaminated bed. To the doctors it may have been a symptom of depression: to her it was a world view. In the absence of any more hopeful 'sense of order', she saw herself as inaccessible to help and unable to help herself.

Respect

Yet, however low Angie's self-esteem, however restricted her mentality by drugs or depression, however confined by poverty or ill-health, however restricted by her position in society, she remains important in herself, a person. This person is as apparent to her as anything else that exists: on some occasions it may appear to be the only reality. Each of us, introspecting, can say the same for ourselves. If we feel at times the victims of circumstance, at the same time we feel to some degree in control of our actions and fates, and revolt against any forces or agents which seek to reduce our powers of self-determination or question our existence as separate individuals. We are not alone in this struggle, yet all our experiences of another person are experiences in part. Some would maintain that it is only through trying to understand others, however hard this can be, that we come to understand ourselves and establish our own identity.

This notion is not an easy one to speak about directly. 'Loving your neighbour as yourself' is such a 'hot' concept as to be uncomfortable, and we rightly distrust anyone who seems to find that such phrases trip easily off the tongue. But in practice, we need such language to understand human behaviour adequately. Dr McVie could have said that family quarrels were nothing to do with him. Geoff and Sheila could have allowed their knowledge of Mr Carter's circumstances to be confined to the immediate causes of his heart attack. Mrs Jarvis could have restricted her interest to Jason's feeding. Their actions imply that they saw their jobs as more than alienated technical exercises. The person of the patient was important.

Once this approach to other people is identified many discussions of morality become clearer. Being truthful, keeping promises, protecting the weak, avoiding harm, respecting dignity: all these are important moral guidelines which derive from our acknowledgement of the intrinsic moral worth of the other person as being equal to our own, an equality demanding of our attention.[2] The difficulty is to deliver respect. We may take it for granted in ordinary living. It is more noticeable when it withers and dies. Why has Angie such a low opinion of herself? Who has shown her adequate respect? Several well-meaning people have tried to help her but she remains 'stuck halfway'. Treated as a child by her parents and Dr McVie when she needed to be an adult, she is now being judged for failing as an adult when she needs room for the child in her to grow up. No one is meeting Angie where she is.

To give true effect to respect, it is the other person's own scale of values, not our own, that we need to enter into. To do this means an attempt at the impossible, to know someone else from the inside. How can we approximate to this?

Attention

'Attention, attention, must be finally paid to such a person', cries Linda in *Death of a Salesman*. No one responds.[3]

Many failures come because of simple inattention. We see everything, we observe so little: we choose to leave out, rather than to include. We prejudge to save time, we become prejudiced. Just another silly teenage overdose: just another unsympathetic doctor. George Orwell describes in *Down and Out in Paris and London* how, when he put on the dirty second-hand clothes of a tramp, he literally disappeared, and people bumped into him in the street.[4] Certain costumes, certain behaviours, make people melt into the background because of visual or verbal clues which say to our mind – 'you need pay no attention here'. The waiter, the shop assistant, the tramp on the road – and, if we're not careful, the patient. 'They used to walk past.' This facet of respect may explain why, in some circumstances, listening is so much more powerful than telling, and caring ignorance better therapy than dismissive authority. The man who pays attention is repaid with interest.

With a complicated problem it is so much easier to accept someone else's version than to check it out ourselves. We often accept in a strange wholesale way political opinions or aesthetic judgements. When it comes to personal relationships, similar forces can be seen at work: we may have formed first impressions of people before we have ever met them, so we do not trouble to re-examine them. Yet this is a marked contrast to some facets of medical work, where a patient with a difficult diagnostic or management problem may be questioned and examined by dozens of professionals in the course of a stay in hospital.

When one's job is dealing with suffering it is often easy to overlook where the pain really lies. Auden realized how much human agony is on the edge of our field of vision, as he stood in front of Brueghel's painting of the *Fall of Icarus*, noting:

how everything turns away
Quite leisurely from the disaster; the ploughman may
Have heard the splash, the forsaken cry,
But for him it was not an important failure; the sun shone
As it had to on the white legs disappearing into the green
Water: and the expensive delicate ship that must have seen
Something amazing, a boy falling out of the sky,
Had somewhere to get to and sailed calmly on.[5]

There is always somewhere to get to, and that is one of the main defences that anyone has against turning aside from well-worn paths. But an emergency operation, a reception into care, sedating a troublesome patient, in themselves take time, and often these things prove to be quite unnecessary if we stop to consider the 'something amazing' that we need to look at. Respecting someone may just mean leaving him or her alone. If we cannot produce solutions, it is always important to be able to offer enough time to listen to the person and hear what is to be told. We cannot ever cross the divide between ourselves and others: but we can pay attention to what they tell us they see on their side.

Empathy

Thus, the way of crossing the gulf between persons must be by using imagination and empathy. When Sheila said to Angie 'I know how you feel', Angie was angry – only later did she realize that Sheila, following her initial meeting with Angie, really had gained insight into some of the things which Angie was facing. Sheila seemed to have responded to the conflicting emotions within Angie's world. But empathy is a subtle and somewhat paradoxical notion. If it becomes a professional technique then it defeats its own purpose: but if it is a genuine sharing in the other's inner world, then the danger is that the helper too will lose bearings and will become engulfed by the client's confusion. Perhaps Angie realized, in rebuffing Sheila, that two drowning souls clinging to a spar which would just about support one, was an obvious disaster.

So empathy points again to that difficult boundary between the professional and the personal, referred to in the previous chapter. In order to stay in that no man's land between professional detachment and personal involvement, we need to be clearer as to what we understand by 'the patient as a person'.

How is such an understanding to be gained? We can point to a number of human capacities to explain what we mean by a person, for example the ability to reason, to communicate with others and to recognize one's own continuing identity. However, none of these descriptions seems to do justice to our common-sense understanding, for each selects a facet of the person, but misses the whole.

The metaphor of dimensions used in the previous chapter

54

has suggested that we can gain a three-dimensional view of others by altering the focal length of our perception or by shifting our perspective in order to see them 'in the round' rather than in a flat two-dimensional way. But this will still be only a view of a static object, neatly labelled, more completely documented, but not a person. For the image to live and move and breathe, we must add time, the fourth dimension: the language of growth, development and change. True morality can only be four-dimensional.

In adding the time dimension we are often limited to the 'snapshot' approach, asking ourselves 'what has changed?' – a series of glimpses of the individual at different stages. This adds movement, but in a flickering, jerky way rather like an old movie. The study of 'passages' or 'life events' takes this approach,[6] but still may not enable us to see a person for what he or she really is, and so protect the personal values which have been demonstrated to be under threat.

Angie and Jason are clearly persons under threat. As Mrs Jarvis listened with sympathy but some bewilderment to Angie's seemingly disconnected ramblings, some patterns began to emerge which she could sense might help her understand Angie as a person. Angie was making links between her present distress and her past experience which obviously carried a special meaning for her, and which in turn would help to shape her future. The quality of Mrs Jarvis's help depends on her ability to recognize these inner connections. She might be drawn out of her bewilderment by paying attention to Angie's history, the relationships she is creating, and her potential for growth.

Having a History

Angie knows herself to be unique because of her awareness, stretching back in time, of a unified succession of experiences she calls 'her life'. She may try to describe this to others like Mrs Jarvis but she alone knows it from within. The sound of her father's laughter, her mother's tense embrace, the feel of Jason's hands are her experiences, and belong to no one else. No impersonal description can make them real.

A person's history is a guide to them in writing, as it were,

55

the next chapter of their lives. But we may now see why professional interventions can threaten the person, because the professional will be used as the author. Rarely is the presumption of writing someone else's case history recognized. In extreme situations, no attempt will be made to discover, in words or through imagination, how the patient might wish to shape his or her future from these previous experiences. Thus the first step is helping a patient like Angie to write her own life history.[7] She alone knows the inside story, how it feels to be her. It is a story she may not want to think about. It may be too full of pain, or of guilt or of unresolved anger at people who have hurt her. She may want to hand the story over to the doctor, nurse or social worker, to let them write the happy ending if they can – repair the damaged love affair, staunch the bleeding womb, treat the overdose, keep her baby safe. But painful or pleasurable, the life history is Angie's, and it can never be given or taken away.

Creating Relationships

Whatever our history, we must live in the present with others around us. Our day-to-day relationships vary greatly in intensity, and we can only sustain a very few close encounters in any given time. Most of our relationships are part of a routine or ritual, and little of us is invested in them, but from them we may move through a range to the closest, most demanding and rewarding. To be a person is to be the creator of and responder to such a range: and the habit which diminishes the flexibility diminishes the person.

Angie was further diminished by her career in hospital after Jason's birth. The danger to personhood occurs when the professional intervention reduces the person to a patient (the person suffering from epilepsy becomes 'an epileptic', the person with a drink problem 'an alcoholic'). It is this move (often a collusion between person and professional helper) which dramatically forecloses the range of relationships originally open to the individual in his or her creativity as a person.

Angie is now, it seems, hovering on the verge of becoming

permanently dependent on others. Voices from the past disable her – 'over my dead body', 'you can't cope', 'you must achieve', 'satisfy *me*'. She has already found that people are willing to 'manage' her if she can express her bewilderment in a problem within their sphere: a sore tummy brings the kindly GP; her obvious anxiety produces tranquillizers; her problems with baby bring the health visitor. Each demand to create or alter a *relationship* can be translated into a specific demand for outside assistance. She is learning fast what it takes to be a patient – and how to stay that way.

There was fleeting contact between Angie and Sheila which might have provided friendship and companionship for Angie. In other circumstances a nurse nearer Angie's age might have got close to her. But Angie was not ready. When Mrs Jarvis visits her, her isolation is obviously increasing, and she is retreating into a private world from which it may be difficult to escape. Angie must begin to build new relationships before health can be restored.

Potential

The third feature of being a person is enshrined in the hopes and fears that each one has for the future, and for continuing change and development of mind and body. At this point in the story, there seems more fear than hope for Angie. After Mr Carter's death, the future looks bleak for her and her mother. Medical workers are prone to see the pathology and problems more clearly than the more hopeful aspects of people's lives, and at times this may be appropriate. Yet such restricted vision is often responsible for one of the most subtle moral failures – the failure to see potential for personal growth even in the worst situations. They fail their patients if by their approach they confirm only the patients' disabilities, infecting them with pessimism and anxiety. Human life can be viewed merely as a decline to death, and medical work as a desperate battle to postpone the inevitable. In a sense this is realism, but a realism which reduces a person to mere physiology. We need not see always 'the skull beneath the skin'.[8]

What is the potential for Angie and her baby? Obviously they both have life before them still, many years in which to grow and develop. The problem is that Angie feels 'stuck' and this may make Jason's voyage a dangerous one. Yet Angie has so much to give, to herself and to her child. She is intelligent, perceptive, independent to a degree and feels things deeply. Her childhood was no worse than most, even if her adolescence is a stormy one. She still sees her parents' love and concern, though distorted through the pain of recent events. She has resources within herself, if only she can be helped to find them. So far, professional helpers appear only to have reacted to crises, to have responded to what *has* happened: no one has helped Angie to look towards what *could* be.

'When will it be me?' asked Angie of Mrs Jarvis. To help answer this question, professionals have to learn to look at their own person and experiences. We each, like Angie, have our own history, present relationships and potential. Previous experiences, unresolved and poorly understood, may alter much that we do, certainly modify how we do it. Why Dr McVie, Sheila, Sister Curran and Mrs Jarvis acted in the restricted way they did needs to be examined – by looking for Angie's potential they might have found their own as well. But sometimes, as has happened with Angie, other people, trying to help, merely inhibit growth. And sometimes things have to get worse before they can get better.

Exercises

1. Group Exercise: To illustrate the difficulties in gaining an understanding of others, split groups into pairs and after ten to fifteen minutes' discussion ask one member of the pair to introduce the other to the whole group by presenting a 'case history'.

2. Role-play can be used to illustrate and explore any aspects of Angie's story, e.g. the visit of Mrs Jarvis can be re-enacted, with different group members trying the part of Angie or of a professional helper. Earlier episodes of the story can be role-played in a similar way, and new characters (e.g. other professional workers) can be added if desired. When role-play is used with a mixed professional group it is useful (and entertaining!) to encourage people to play members of professions other than their own. (It should be stressed that role-play is not acting, and that people are free to use Angie's story as a 'jumping-off point' for recalling similar incidents in their own professional experience, in which the moral issues were difficult to identify and to resolve.)

3. In *A Fortunate Man* John Berger describes disillusionment among doctors in the following terms:

> One of the fundamental reasons why so many doctors become cynical or disillusioned is precisely because, when abstract idealism has worn thin, they are uncertain about the value of the actual lives of the patients they are treating. It is not because they are callous or personally inhuman: it is because they live in and accept a society which is incapable of knowing what human life is worth.

Do you agree with this view?

4. Professional relationships are often caricatured in fiction, but such caricature may reveal important facets of the truth. What can one learn from the following examples about the problems of treating patients as persons?

(a) *The Big Nurse*
The Big Nurse tends to get real put out if something keeps her outfit from running like a smooth, accurate, precision-made machine. The slightest thing messy or out of kilter or in the way ties her into a little white knot of tight-smiled fury. She walks around with that same doll smile crimped between her chin and her nose and that same calm whir coming from her eyes, but down inside

of her she's tense as steel. I know, I can feel it. And she don't relax a hair till she gets the nuisance attended to – what she calls 'adjusted to surroundings'.

And I've watched her get more and more skilful over the years. Practice has steadied and strengthened her until now she wields a sure power that extends in all directions on hairlike wires too small for anybody's eye but mine.

What she dreams of there in the centre of those wires is a world of precision efficiency and tidiness like a pocket watch with a glass back, a place where the schedule is unbreakable and all the patients who aren't Outside, obedient under her beam, are wheelchair Chronics with catheter tubes run direct from every pantleg to the sewer under the floor. Year by year she accumulates her ideal staff: doctors, all ages and types, come and rise up in front of her with ideas of their own about the way a ward should be run, some with backbone enough to stand behind their ideas, and she fixes these doctors with dry-ice eyes day in, day out, until they retreat with unnatural chills. 'I tell you I don't know what it is,' they tell the guy in charge of personnel. 'Since I started on that ward with that woman I feel like my veins are running ammonia. I shiver all the time, my kids won't sit in my lap, my wife won't sleep with me. I *insist* on a transfer – neurology bin, the alky tank, paediatrics, I just don't *care!*'

(K. Kesey, *One Flew Over the Cuckoo's Nest*, Picador, 1973, p. 27)

(b) *'You're very upset'*
Gillian Boyle is 'thirty-five, attractive, and very professional in her manner.' She is a medical social worker.

Mrs Boyle: Good morning.
Ken: Morning.
Mrs Boyle: Mr Harrison?
Ken: (cheerfully) It used to be
Mrs Boyle: My name is Mrs Boyle.
Ken: And you've come to cheer me up.
Mrs Boyle: I wouldn't put it like that.
Ken: How would you put it?
Mrs Boyle: I've come to see if I can help.
Ken: Good. You can.
Mrs Boyle: How?
Ken: Go and convince Dr Frankenstein that he has successfully made his monster and he can now let it go.

Mrs Boyle: Dr Emerson is a first-rate physician. My goodness, they have improved this room.

Ken: Have they?

Mrs Boyle: It used to be really dismal. All dark green and cream. It's surprising what pastel colours will do, isn't it? Really cheerful.

Ken: Yes; perhaps they should try painting me. I'd hate to be the thing that ruins the decor.

As the conversation proceeds, and Ken's frustrations make him more bitter:

Ken: It's marvellous you know.

Mrs Boyle: What is?

Ken: All you people have the same technique. When I say something really awkward you just pretend I haven't said anything at all. You're all the bloody same. . . Well there's another outburst. That should be your cue to comment on the light-shade or the colour of the walls.

Mrs Boyle: I'm sorry if I have upset you.

Ken: Of course you have upset me. You and the doctors with your appalling so-called professionalism, which is nothing more than a series of verbal tricks to prevent you relating to your patients as human beings.

Mrs Boyle: You must understand; we have to remain relatively detached in order to help. . .

Ken: That's alright with me. Detach yourself. Tear yourself off on the dotted line that divides the woman from the social worker and post yourself off to another patient.

Mrs Boyle: You're very upset. . .

Ken: Christ Almighty, you're doing it again. Listen to yourself woman. I say something offensive about you and you turn your professional cheek. If you were human, if you were treating me as human, you'd tell me to bugger off. Can't you see that this is why I've decided that life isn't worth living? I am not human and I'm even more convinced of that by your visit than I was before, so how does that grab you? The very exercise of your so-called *professionalism* makes me want to die.

(From Brian Clark
Whose Life is it Anyway?
(Amber Lane Press, 1978))

5. Explore the attitudes to the dying person which the following extract from Tolstoy's *The Death of Ivan Ilyich* reveals:

What tormented Ivan Ilyich most was the pretence, the lie, which for some reason they all kept up, that he was merely ill and not dying, and that he only need stay quiet and carry out the doctor's orders, and then some great change for the better would result. But *he* knew that whatever they might do nothing would come of it except still more agonizing suffering and death. And the pretence made him wretched: it tormented him that they refused to admit what they knew and he knew to be a fact, but persisted in lying to him concerning his terrible condition, and wanted him and forced him to be a party to the lie. Deceit, this deceit enacted over him up to the very eve of his death: this lying which could only degrade the awful, solemn act of his death to the level of their visitings, their curtains, their sturgeon for dinner . . . was horribly painful to Ivan Ilyich. And it was a strange thing – many a time when they were playing their farce for his benefit he was within a hair's breadth of shouting at them: 'Stop lying! You know, and I know, that I am dying. So do at least stop lying about it!' But he had never had the spirit to do it. The awful, terrible act of his dying was, he saw, reduced by those about him to the level of a fortuitous, disagreeable and rather indecent incident (much in the same way as people behave with someone who goes into a drawing-room smelling unpleasantly) – and this was being done in the name of the very decorum he had served all his life long. He saw that no one felt for him, because no one was willing even to appreciate his situation.

(The *Death of Ivan Ilyich*, Penguin
Books, 1960, pp. 142f)

5

Relations

Social Service departments come in two sorts – the ones equipped in the fat years, and those set up in the lean. This was one of the latter. The Council had clearly had to spend some money fast the previous year, and so the long corridor at least had been redecorated: but the improvements were not enough to reassure Mrs Carter. To her these places had always seemed like where the other people go, the ones who never make preparations, and get them wrong when they do. For those who think ahead, like Mrs Carter, thought had never encompassed places like this – not for family matters, not in a thousand years. That's why she had phoned first.

Suddenly it all seemed a terrible mistake. Loyalty was more important. They had never been in trouble like this before, even when things went so wrong and John had been drinking so much. Even then, working hard to wrap up the bottles, collecting him, coping with the boss, getting him to the clinic, Mrs Carter had managed without anyone else knowing. It had worked then hadn't it? Why wouldn't that work now – even John would have agreed. Turn round, turn round, it's not too late.

She paused and began to turn on her heel.

'It is too late. I've let the cat out of the bag' she thought. 'Something has to be done – I said that. Neighbours have noticed, and there was that police incident. Anyway, Jason is more than my pride, isn't he? Jason.'

She kept repeating his name to keep her walking past the bicycles and the pram towards the glass window at the inquiry desk.

The phone rang as she reached the window and it made her jump. Someone else like her, ringing in to tell tales. She looked around as if expecting a man in a dark overcoat.

'And what if Angie were coming here today? She has been put in touch with them by that health visitor, I know.' Her hand paused on the button by the window.

'It's all for the best really, for Angie and Jason. That's what the social worker had said. He is right too.' He – funny how she'd expected a woman, and had wanted someone her own age who had been through it, who would understand. He sounded as if he might try to understand, but he didn't seem much older than Angie herself.

'I've come to see, er, Mr Jackson. Yes, he is expecting me. I'll wait here.'

'He should be anyway,' she thought, 'after all the fuss I've created. Something does need to be done. Angie is a different girl since she's been in that flat. She won't ring me, won't invite me, almost won't let me in when I call, even when the neighbours ask me to go round. They said the police had called the day before, bringing Jason back after he had been left outside the supermarket. Angie didn't tell me, but the neighbours thought the police had been very kind. It all could have been a mistake, but the crying that they'd told me about wasn't. Four hours they said Jason had been crying, four hours.

'Four hours. That was the time they had heard, but how much longer was it really? It had taken an age for Angie to come to the door. She'd got straight out of bed. I thought she'd taken an overdose again but there weren't any signs of it. Too tired to get up, is that really what she'd said?

'She certainly looked it.'

'God, why am I left alone to cope with all this? Hasn't there been enough already? First the rows about sex, the heavy drinking, the hushing it all up away from the neighbours and away from Angie. Then there was that thing in my breast – a shock, but being half a woman at least kept him at bay. He did his best I suppose. A man's a man after all. He was always terribly kind to Angie – he'd do anything for her, take her places, fetch her at all hours, comfort her, get up in the night with her monster dreams. "Mr Softy" – it had been a joke at first anyway. I suppose in a way it made up for *us*. Oh John, John, why did you leave me?

'I knew Angie hadn't fed Jason. His nappy was wringing wet too. But wet enough to cause blisters like that? Oh John.'

She hadn't heard the door open.

'Thank you for coming Mrs Carter. Would you like to come this way?'

A very kind voice. Not looking much older than Angie, she was right. But then they're all like that, aren't they?

'Something's got to be done!' Mrs Carter's plea is likely to cause a spasm of guilt and antagonism in the people who have been trying to help Angie so far. Have they overlooked something? Is the whole thing going to turn nasty, with perhaps charges of professional incompetence or worse? Or is this just the cry of an over-anxious and possessive mother who cannot stop trying to manage her daughter's life? When the spectre of baby battering is raised, these questions become urgent. Somehow a balance has to be found between necessary intervention for the baby's sake and unwarranted interference initiated by the grandmother.

The dilemma provoked by Mrs Carter illustrates the problem of defining the limits of the rights of individuals, and of deciding how such rights fit in to a wider social morality. John Donne's much quoted words 'no man is an island' are balanced by Jean-Paul Sartre's, 'Hell is other people'.[1] We are not isolated individuals. We live within a complex network of interpersonal relationships and this network can support us or ensnare us. A weakness of much discussion about medical ethics is that it tends to ignore the social dimension, dealing with every problem as though it were just a private matter between individual patient and individual practitioner, and this point of view is taken by most professional codes of ethics. Such an approach has great strengths. It can provide a protection for personal values and the autonomy of individuals. But it is not the whole story. The relations between people, the extent of their obligations to one another, the conflicts between one person's rights and another's – such issues are raised in daily encounters between practitioner and patient. We might try to ignore them, but that will not make them go away.

Let us look at the different levels of relationship in which Angie is involved. Those with greatest intensity might be loosely described as 'family'. Her son, Jason, her mother, her dead father and her absent boyfriend, all affect her in important ways. She feels the ties of love and dependence, but also the pain of anger and guilt. Her relationship with her parents seems particularly troubled, giving her little foundation on which to build a stable relationship with her boyfriend and her baby. Perhaps Philip Larkin's bitter words would fit Angie:

They fuck you up, your mum and dad.
  They may not mean to, but they do.
They fill you with the faults they had
  And add some extra just for you.

But they were fucked up in their turn
  By fools in old-style hats and coats,
Who half the time were soppy-stern
  And half at one another's throats.[2]

At a less intense level Angie has accumulated relationships
with various professional helpers. There is Dr McVie, the
fatherly GP, who has known her since she was a little girl and
perhaps still sees her as such. There are the hospital staff who
met her when Jason was born, who worried about her in
passing, but are not now in a position to help. There is Mrs
Jarvis, warm and motherly, a mixture of professional health
visitor and friend. Now a social worker is being called into
the scene, apparently an emissary from mother, who will have
to persuade Angie that he isn't taking sides. None of these
relationships is particularly close, but with Angie's small family and lack of friends, any one of them could become important to her if a crisis develops.

More distant again are what can vaguely be called relationships with 'society'. Largely an unseen presence, the society still affects Angie in numerous ways – the character of
the neighbourhood in which she lives, the values communi-
cated in the press and on television, the regulations which
allocate her social security payments, the policies which determine whether she will be re-housed. Perhaps for Angie
society is rather like a sleeping monster, but it will awaken if
her behaviour becomes too bizarre or if she does assault her
baby.

These three levels of relationship – with family, professional
helpers and society – each has its own moral problems. For
society it is the problem of the limits of individual freedom;
for the professions it is the problem of defining responsibility;
for the family, it is the problem of love and duty. We shall
look at each in turn, in relation to Angie and to other patients.

Limits to Freedom

It is obvious that society imposes limits of all kinds on the behaviour of its individual members, ranging from the subtle influence of convention to the precise requirements of law. Such limits are not necessarily destructive of individual freedom. Freedom should not be equated with letting everyone do whatever they choose. A society without controls on behaviour would merely put the weak at the mercy of the strong and would create a perpetual state of chaos and fear. The problem is to get the right balance between freedom and control. Too much control ignores or represses individual initiative and creativity – too little opens the gates to injustice and exploitation.

For someone like Angie, the society may seem a faceless and alien force. Perhaps she feels that most of the time the neighbours just don't want to know, but let her step out of line, act a little strangely and they'll soon be talking about her behind her back. She may feel the same about the authorities. What do they care about her struggle to manage in an unsuitable house with no husband and only social security? But let them think she's harming Jason and they're on to her like a ton of bricks. Why can't they just leave her alone?

This sense of conflict between the individual in trouble and society is very common, and there seems no obvious way of overcoming it. Frequently all that seems possible is recourse to the law, to prevent people damaging themselves or others, even though this leaves the basic problem unsolved:

Rondo, a young black man of 23, a poor achiever at school and constantly in trouble with the police, began to act strangely, and to be violent towards his family. A number of psychiatrists, seeing him in prison or in hospital, declared that he was not suffering from a formal mental illness, and he could not be admitted against his will to a psychiatric hospital, nor was there much to be gained from informal admission, should he ever agree to this. At home, he continued to behave violently, possibly under the influence of drugs he obtained himself. The probation officer and the local priest of the church where the family attended called in the GP. Because of the pyschiatrist's views, no medical action could be taken, and the young man eventually was arrested and returned to prison.[3]

Rondo's progress from prison and back again illustrates the limits of law. We frequently speak of the 'force of law'. It is an appropriate phrase, because an important feature of all legal intervention is that it can be backed up by physical force if necessary. Thus the law is (or should be) an effective defender of the weaker members of society, protecting them against exploitation and loss of rights. Yet the very force of the law makes it a rather clumsy instrument when we are dealing with the subtler aspects of human relationships. We see this in the case of Rondo. The Mental Health Act did not, in the psychiatrist's judgement, apply to him and so he could not be kept in psychiatric hospital, where he might have been helped to modify his violent behaviour. Once he was at home, no one seemed able to avert his collision course with the criminal law, which merely returned him to prison. Thus the best the law could do was to stop Rondo causing harm. There seemed to be no legal means of providing him with positive help.

If Angie is injuring her baby, then the same problem will arise. The law quite rightly provides protection for the child. Perhaps Jason will have to be removed from his mother and put into local authority care. But again this forcible legal intervention will merely prevent further harm. It will not heal the wounds in Angie's life which are causing her strange behaviour. It will not give Jason the mother he needs.

In view of this, it is not surprising that most doctors and social workers invoke legal means only as the very last resort, hoping that people like Rondo and Angie can be helped by voluntary measures before they do cause harm to themselves or to others. Legally enforced intervention is often seen as a professional failure or even an evasion of responsibility by those who are supposed to be the patient's helpers and allies. But in fact such interventions are rarely the fault of the professional helpers, who can hardly be expected to change overnight the kind of problems which Angie and Rondo face. The fault lies with the society as a whole.

Why is it that social problems like juvenile violence and

baby battering seem so intractable? Attempts to answer this question move the debate out of the sphere of the criminal law and into the political area, where issues of priorities in government expenditure and in general social policy arise. Why does so much money and effort go into healing the injuries which Rondo and Angie may cause, but so little into understanding and changing the conditions which cause their violent behaviour? How could social conditions be altered so that people feel supported and understood, not alienated and rejected?

Such problems seem so intractable that most people abandon attempts to think out solutions. One might have thought that health care professionals, dealing daily with society's casualties, would be motivated to try to discover and correct some of the causes. (They are hardly likely to do themselves out of a job in the near future!) Yet there is great hesitation in the professions to becoming too closely involved with political and social issues. This is based partly on a fear that the much prized autonomy of the professions could be threatened if they became too politically assertive and partly on the feeling that such issues are really outside professional competence and people disagree about how they should be tackled. Yet socio-political involvement can take many forms. Increasingly, doctors, nurses and social workers are seeing that part of their responsibility is to effect political change through influencing public opinion. Voluntary associations and campaigns concerned with a wide range of issues – alcohol abuse, cigarette smoking, terminal care, housing, nuclear policy, the handicapped and many others – offer opportunities for professional expertise and experience to help change society. It is a matter of finding how to change the limits which diminish and threaten people into boundaries within which they can find freedom.

Authority and Responsibility

Within the narrower circle of relationships between Angie and the doctors, nurses, health visitor and social worker who tried to help her, there arises a new set of issues. Let us recall Angie's quite varied career as a patient. Her story begins with a physical symptom, but one without obvious cause. This brings her into the domain of the GP, but leaves a question mark over his ability to help her, apart from immediate symptom relief. Her next encounter with the health service is in the role of bereaved relative and this is perfunctory and inconclusive. Her pregnancy brings her into more clearly defined relationships with both community and hospital services, yet the extent to which she needs more extensive help is difficult to estimate. Thereafter as a young mother who does not seem to be coping well she is given support and advice by a health visitor and a social worker. Finally, as her behaviour causes increasing concern, the likelihood of psychiatric referral emerges, and since her behaviour may indicate a psychiatric illness[4], her problems begin to take on a medical aspect once more. Many people follow similar courses to Angie's, moving from episodes of relatively serious upset to periods of minor disturbance and unhappiness, encountering several different kinds of health worker *en route*. The question is, how can such a variety of helping relationships most benefit the patient?

We can try to answer the question by considering the *authority* and the *responsibility*[5] of the various professions involved in health care. Both of these terms can be used in a variety of senses. In the case of authority we can distinguish between authority based on knowledge (sapiential authority), authority based on personality (charismatic authority) and authority based on social role (ascribed authority). Ideally all three types of authority coalesce in any individual case: we hope that people are fitted to the social role ascribed to them both in terms of their personality attributes and in terms of the knowledge they possess. In reality, however, people in positions of authority do not always possess the desired personality traits or knowledge. A nurse administrator, a medical consultant, a senior social worker may lack an up-to-date knowledge of their field or may fail to command respect. Nevertheless (except in cases of gross incompetence) it is necessary to allow them the authority of their position in order to keep the health care system functioning. The situation becomes much more complicated however when several different professions are involved in the care of one individual.

Clearly each profession has its own sapiential authority and can claim priority when aspects of the case which fall within their field are being discussed. But, of course, patients are not neatly parcelled into bits corresponding to the different professional interests, and in any case one profession will often carry out 'border raids' into the other's territory, as the following incident illustrates:

> Mrs Buxton, an elderly lady living alone, was becoming more and more immobile. She was attended by a trainee general practitioner and a young social worker, both new to the area. The trainee GP thought that, if more social service support were to be provided, the old lady could manage at home, and rang the Home Help Office to arrange this. The social worker, shocked by the home conditions, felt that the old lady should be admitted to the local geriatric ward, but could not persuade the GP to do this. The old lady herself just pottered on, until she teetered on the edge of a mat and toppled over. In her fall, she hurt her leg. Without consulting the doctor, the social worker had the old lady admitted to hospital by emergency ambulance.[6]

There was a lot of 'border raiding' in this case, with each professional trying to do the other one's job! How should the trainee GP and the social worker have co-operated in helping Mrs Buxton?

An answer may lie in clarifying the nature of professional responsibility. Like authority, responsibility can be used in several different senses. To be responsible is to be 'answerable' – but answerable to whom about what? In its narrowest sense responsibility refers to legal liability. For example, when a patient is admitted to hospital it is customary for one consultant to be in charge of the case. This means that, in the event of a legal action for damages, both the consultant and the health authority may be liable. Legal responsibility is less clearly defined when the patient is not in hospital. If a patient were being seen by a general practitioner, a health visitor and a social worker, no one professional would be regarded as having overall responsibility in a legal sense. (An exception to this is when a court makes an order placing specific legal responsibilities on social workers for care and supervision.) But responsibility can be extended beyond legal liability. A person can *feel* responsible, even though the law may not hold him or her responsible. For example, general practitioners regard themselves as responsible for the continuity of care of their patients. This is recognized by the National Health Service in its practice of allowing access to specialists only through general practitioners and requiring that information about a patient gained in hospital be passed on to the patient's own general practitioner on his return home. Social workers also feel this sense of general responsibility for their clients and may seek to gain as full a picture as possible of their social and medical history, though this is less easy for them than it is for the GP because of the confidentiality attached to medical records.

Wider still than legal and professional responsibility is moral responsibility. This is a concern with answering not the law or the expectations of one's profession, but the inner commitment which leads many people into the health care professions. Could I have helped the person more? Patients often fall through the gaps in the system. No one is guilty of malpractice or of a lack of professionalism and yet the person has not been helped.

To help any individual patient each professional needs as rich an understanding as possible, which can be gained by an openness to the quite different insights into the problem gained by members of other professions. In Mrs Buxton's case, the social worker acted wrongly, not by calling an ambulance (any neighbour might have done that), but by using the old lady's accident to out-manoeuvre the patient's GP, just as the doctor had earlier tried to arrange social work help behind her back. It is when professionals refuse to communicate properly with one another or when they compete with one another to make their own view prevail that patients become the victims of professionalism. When responsibility for helping the patient is shared, with no one profession insisting on its omnicompetence and infallibility, there is a better chance that the individuality of the patient will be respected and the appropriate form of help given.

Family Love and Duty

Perhaps, if society neglects and professionals misinterpret people's needs, the family at least will understand. Yet understanding seemed a major difficulty in the Carter family, and this is not uncommon especially between generations, as the following case illustrates:

Mrs Dent was an elderly lady who had developed severe heart failure for which major diuretic therapy was needed. Without the treatment she was extremely distressed and breathless, but whatever regime was tried in treatment, she had difficulty with continence. Never very clean in her habits, she often failed to reach the lavatory or commode in time. She lived on the ground floor of a house, leased in her name, while her daughter-in-law and son lived with their family on the upper floor, on a separate lease, but with common access to the street. They cooked every meal for her and dealt with most of her ordinary needs.

The old lady was also cared for by the district nurse, received meals on wheels at lunchtime and was content and happy to be in her home. Every time she had a major episode of incontinence, however, the family upstairs tried to press her and the nurse and the doctors, to 'get her away'. The old lady refused to go to hospital under any circumstances. The family approached the hospital out-patient department, the community health services, and they wrote strong letters to the family doctor. The children in the family were brought with physical and psychological symptoms to the family doctor, who also looked after the old lady. The parents always stressed that the root of the problem lay 'in the conditions we are forced to live in'. Rehousing offers were turned down: it was the old lady who 'had to go'.

The house was indeed extremely smelly, but the nurse and the doctor, in discussing the situation with the old lady, were unable to change her views, and felt that, since she was being offered every facility at home, they were doing their duty. Strenuous attempts to try to unravel the reason for such bitterness between the generations also failed. Finally, the old lady caught pneumonia and was persuaded by the nurse to allow herself to be admitted to hospital, where she died peacefully. The family continued to be angry, and accused the practice of failing to care for their mother adequately.[7]

It is interesting to note that in this case the doctor and nurse in acting as the patient's advocates found themselves opposing the family. They could also sympathize with the family's point of view. Caring for the old lady was not an easy or a pleasant task. Yet the family could not see what was so obvious to the professional helpers – that staying in her own home was of vital importance to the old person to maintain her sense of worth and dignity. The relatives were too close to the incompetent aspects of Mrs Dent's behaviour to be able to see her any more as an independent person with her own needs and values. Incontinence is a particularly demeaning aspect of ageing. It rapidly lowers one's status in other people's eyes, making one into a case to be managed, a mess to be tidied up.

This lack of understanding between close relatives is not unusual. Angie and her mother shared the shock of sudden bereavement, but seemed powerless to help one another. Could Angie recognize the losses her mother had known – the near tragedy of Angie's difficult birth, the trauma of mastectomy, the death of a husband, the leaving home of her young daughter and now fears of injury to her grandson? It seemed not. Yet equally Mrs Carter seemed insensitive to her daughter's suffering. Did she remember how she had failed to support her against her father's anger? Could she understand how hard it was for Angie, now that the boyfriend had deserted her, to admit that perhaps she had made a mistake? Could she see that her seeming hardness and efficiency as a housewife and mother made Angie even more depressed and unsure of herself? Apparently not. The closeness of family relationships, which can provide great support, can also blind people to one another's needs. The pain they feel obscures the pain they cause.

Despite the difficulties, however, it is such close personal relationships that hold the greatest significance for an individual's health and well-being. The tragedy for the old lady insisting on staying at home was that she held on to her independence at the cost of her family's love. Her family cared for her out of a sense of duty, but their anger smouldered underneath, venting itself after her death on the doctor and the nurse. Something similar seems to be happening to Angie. She too has her independence, her home and her baby, but the heritage of anger and violence from her unresolved relationships at home now threatens Jason. The healing of Angie must involve the healing of her relationships, for they underlie so much of her physical and emotional distress.

'Something's got to be done' said Mrs Carter on the telephone to the social worker. The problem is that what's got to be done needs to be spontaneous. It is the familiar paradox of love and duty. A mother has a duty to care for her baby, but an essential part of that care is maternal warmth and affection. These aspects of mothering cannot be commanded. They are natural responses which the child senses in the mother's body. We might be tempted to reply to Mrs Carter, 'Be more relaxed with Angie and things might improve.' But again *ordering* someone to relax is as pointless as ordering someone to be affectionate. Our instruction will probably make them still less relaxed. ('Don't be nervous', says the King of Hearts to the Mad Hatter in *Alice in Wonderland*, 'or I'll have you executed on the spot.')

A solution may lie in recognizing that professional helping relationships can be useful as temporary substitutes for inadequate family relationships. The kindly doctor and nurse who backed up the old lady in her wish to stay at home were offering themselves as the sympathetic children she failed to find in her own family. (Unfortunately they were unable to pass this role on to the real children, hard as they tried.) Dr McVie acted the understanding father to Angie, and Mrs Jarvis the warm mother. Angie turned to them as much for emotional as for medical help. (Sheila, the house physician, almost became a big sister to Angie, but didn't quite know how.) These quasi-familial relationships offered by professional helpers should not become *permanent* substitutes for the real relationships. When this happens we have the symbiotic relationship of parental helper and dependent patient, which cannot lead to health, because the relationship is self-perpetuating. (The game of 'Stay sick, I need you'.)[8] They should provide bridges back to the more painful and complex relationships in the family, where the hurt has been caused in the first place. It is a waste of time to *tell* people to relax or to be loving, but our acts of helping can *show* them and encourage them to try for themselves.

Sharing

Our aim throughout this chapter has been to encourage a broader view of the patient's life than that which stresses only individuality and inner states. Each individual person discovers his or her individuality by relating to others, discovering points in common and points of individual difference. Often society and family seem to bring more harm than benefit, yet without them the person could have no sense of identity, no way of defining purposes and goals. Professional intervention may at times mean advocacy for the individual's rights against threats from outside, but just as frequently it entails putting the patient back in touch with social reality. Recovery means return to a place (perhaps a new place) in the family and the wider society.

In order to assist in this way professional helpers must themselves learn social skills. Traditionally professionals are accustomed to being independent practitioners, in control of a situation or playing a clearly defined role within it. They find shared responsibility difficult and seem to lack an adequate language for communicating across professional boundaries. Often they fear a loss of power or status if they admit to inadequacies or a feeling of helplessness to colleagues, most especially if those colleagues are in a different profession.

A group of professional trainees were divided into two groups and set an exercise in group co-operation. Each person had a set of pieces from which he was required to make a square. Since no one had the correct set it was necessary for group members to exchange pieces until the sets made up squares. No speech or sign language was allowed. Instead each person had to notice whether he had

76

a piece needed by someone else and to pass it over without being asked.

One group completed the exercise in a few minutes, but the second group was still unable to finish after nearly half an hour. Subsequent discussion revolved round what had happened in the second group and on the feelings of helplessness, frustration and anger in its members.[9]

Exercises of this type can alert people to the basic attitudes required, if sharing is to take place. Even although the exercise may appear somewhat contrived, it has an obvious application to interprofessional co-operation. Often appropriate help cannot be given to people in need until the various people trying to help are willing to share their insights (including their feelings of inability to help) and to see what another needs. Getting together over a case can produce a solution which no one person can find unaided. Of course, sharing is required with the patient or client as well. There may be a need for a much more adventurous approach to case conferences than the present practice. Why is it that the patient is excluded, or allowed in only as a person to be interrogated and demonstrated upon before the discussion?

In addition to the change of attitudes required in order to improve sharing between professionals and between professionals and their patients, there is a need to look more carefully at how they communicate. Finding a common language must mean thinking about the 'rules of the game', which distinguish a good argument from a bad one and which help people understand one another's viewpoint. In the next chapter we shall look at the ways people can learn to improve their communication, using the context of an interprofessional case conference, where decisions must be backed up by reasons.

Exercises

1. The death from parental injuries of seven-year-old Maria Colwell in 1974 raised public awareness of the extent of child abuse and of the dilemmas it provokes for professional agencies. A report by the local authority responsible for Maria at the time made numerous recommendations designed to avert similar tragedies. Among them was the need for change of professional attitudes to confidentiality. The Director of Social Services stated:

> It is right that privacy of information about individuals should be treated as of the utmost importance, but it can be an obstacle to reaching an informed decision about a child at risk.
> But where there is mutual trust and understanding between the professions involved, confidentiality should cease to be an issue.
>
> (*Daily Telegraph*, 30 April 1975)

Discuss (a) the moral issue raised by the Director's statement; and (b) whether the solution he suggests is adequate.

2. A paediatrician was recently accused of the attempted murder of a Down's Syndrome baby by prescribing a sedative analgesic and ordering nursing care only. After he was acquitted the following joint statement was issued by the British Medical Association, the Royal College of Nursing and the Medical Protection Society (November 1981):

> It is the parents who have the responsibility for deciding what is best for their child, but it is the doctor's job to help and advise them, working with the nurses and the rest of the medical team.

Is this an adequate statement of the various responsibilities, in a situation where a decision has been taken that a baby should not be helped to survive?

3. Discuss the moral issues arising in the following case reported by a psychiatrist, with particular reference to three questions:
(1) Were the patient's rights infringed?
(2) Did the psychiatrist fulfil his professional obligations?
(3) Does the fact that the patient settled happily into hospital and seemed to improve after treatment justify the action taken by the family?

A volunteer by family choice

I was asked by a GP a few weeks ago, on a Sunday afternoon, to go and see a patient whom he had been called to see twice during that weekend. She was 70 years old, recently discharged from a general hospital, where she had been complaining that her bowels were not moving. She had other hypochondriacal symptoms. At home she talked incessantly, moved about the house in an agitated manner and was accusing her husband of all sorts of infidelities, etc. (Her husband was 72 and they had been married a year!) Her ceaseless and disconnected talk was getting her husband down. Even her children, who had been initially unsympathetic toward him now supported the old man in the view that something had to be done. The GP had tried to manage with sedatives but the old lady refused to take them. When I arrived her three children plus their spouses and the old man were present, with the old lady lying on the couch. I diagnosed hypomania and believed the situation could be contained by the use of appropriate drugs.

We talked in the kitchen and I suggested my treatment plan, which would avoid hospitalization, but the family by then had no faith in medicines. The patient didn't want to go into hospital: the relatives wanted hospital admission. Although elated and over talkative the patient had not lost her capacity to reason and was in touch with reality. I did not therefore feel that certification was justified. I was also concerned about the effect of such a step on her relationship with the staff once in hospital, and perhaps on her long-term views of her family. When I demurred at compulsory admission, but said I would like her to come voluntarily, the family simply bundled her into one of their cars and took her to the hospital. Once there she willingly stayed and quickly improved with treatment and has been able to return home to her husband.

Was this a miscarriage of the law? – for this was far from voluntary hospitalization. The relatives took the law into their own hands. Was this assault? Should she also have been made a compulsory patient, or was the good-humoured relatives' treatment best? There was the pressure of the social situation. I was quite clear myself that we should try home treatment first, but the home situation did not allow it. There were other pressures too – the time of the day, the demand for an objective medical opinion, simply to support one already made in the family, the attitude of GP, family, husband. I might have found sufficient evidence of derangement to satisfy the Sheriff, but in psychiatry it is important to maintain the relationship of trust with the patient and to put someone on a compulsory order can be very damaging to that relationship.

(See *Journal of Medical Ethics*, vol. vi, no. 1, March 1980, pp.35–40 for a full discussion of this case.)

4. In the light of what you have read so far, consider the medical or social problem of each member of the Carter family in turn from your own viewpoint. If each were to approach you to discuss his or her own problem, are there any factors you should consider in each case which might enable you or compel you to break professional confidence and share the information you had received with a third party?

6

Reasons

Doctor McVie gathered his coat quickly once the case conference was over. He was a bit bored, very hungry and the habits of a busy lifetime were hard to drop. Although the discussion had been friendly and relaxed he never felt easy doing his work like this, reaching conclusions in public rather than privately beside the desk or the bed. He felt uneasy. Had the right decision been made?

'It's not easy working like this, is it doctor?' Mrs Jarvis's voice behind the coat rack seemed to be speaking his own thoughts.

'No. Hang on – your sleeve is inside out. It all seems to be back to front to me, choosing a line of treatment before we're quite sure what the problem really is. I must admit, though, we've been caught unawares. Perish the thought, but with Jason obviously ill and in hospital, or Angie clearly 'sectionable', it would all be very much easier. But thank goodness things aren't so bad as that though I suppose they might become so. How did you think it went?'

'It always takes me a bit of time to separate what we've decided from how we decided it. I am never satisfied about how I manage to put across the health visitor's views in discussions like this. That may seem terribly egocentric, but I still get a slightly panicky feeling each time I have to open my mouth even after all these years at the game! Perhaps it's lack of lunch – don't you have time for a bite at that quiet pub round the back – behind the post office?'

Mr Jackson, the social worker, had come up. 'Do you mind if I join you? It's really so good to put a face to the voices I meet over the phone. I'm sure patients won't want to see either of you over lunchtime.'

Dr McVie laughed. 'I was once asked to wait in the vestibule while the Duchess finished her whisky, egg and milk – but that was a long time ago as a fresh-faced and totally broke young locum! But times have changed. This one's on me now.'

They picked their way through the traffic and were relieved to find the bar almost empty.

'I hope I didn't seem to be too critical of the medical services', said Mr Jackson. 'Thank you – a pint of real ale please. We've all been left rather unhappy haven't we, and I think I was being a bit strident trying to put my own point across. I somehow feel that now the Carter family has asked us for help, if we could have given it without involving an admission we could have worked on helping them all to get together again. Now I'm worried that the opposite will happen. When they are so proud, and we are so busy, a family like this gets less good care than it should anyway from our Department, I think.'

'Well, we're all feeling a little guilty – I certainly am', said Mrs Jarvis. 'There is so much routine work with the new borns at the moment, and we're two below strength in this patch already. Still we all felt at the practice that with support and medication we could get Angie through – and if I were back there now I think I would say the same. Thank goodness I at least have the others at the surgery to discuss it with – so many health visitors have to face decisions like this on their own, and that makes a solitary job dangerously lonely.'

'Well, guilt is out of place, Mrs J. – you've done everything you could. We can't be there every day to make sure she takes the pills.' Dr McVie felt more human with half a cheese sandwich inside him. 'I have to admit I don't find it easy going over and over the same ideas and not seeming to get anywhere. Although the Chairman did very well, it did seem to take an inordinate amount of time to reach an unsatisfactory conclusion. I want to keep Angie home, don't misunderstand me, but as things are now I know we can't manage her *and* be sure that Jason's OK. If she would only allow her mother to look after him – but since she has said to me when I saw her that she would only consider going into hospital if Jason *wasn't* with her mother, we have no choice. Taking the child into care isn't a very satisfactory answer, but it's the only alternative.'

Mr Jackson was going to reply, but thought better of it. Mrs Jarvis broke the silence. 'I know that when Angie is less depressed I can get through to her. The risk is undoubtedly there at the moment – as that policeman kept on saying. It's funny, isn't it, how one reacts to what people are, rather than what they really say. Although he was being perfectly calm and kind, some of us just couldn't think straight about what he was saying, just because he was a policeman. Perhaps it's the same when doctors get together, or nurses for that matter, and seem to "gang up" against the rest.

It took a bit of time for the psychiatrist to come out to meet us halfway, I felt – he was so obsessed by the technicalities of the diagnosis that he didn't seem to see it as a *situation*. It was almost as if we spoke a different language.'

'Hmm. Two nations divided by their common language', mused Dr McVie, misquoting happily.

'Still, many psychiatrists would not have responded so willingly to taking a patient into hospital without an order, so it's a relief that he sees it that way. If only we had a mother and baby unit in the area.'

Mr Jackson's feelings finally surfaced. 'I'm so unhappy about splitting up Jason and Angie, so soon after they have been brought together – the birth must have been such a dreadful time for Angie. It seems to me that we are just compounding their problems, not solving them. It's good in the short term – but what of the time ahead?'

'Well, unsatisfactory as it is, there are the choices, I'm afraid', said Dr McVie. 'We all want the best for the whole family. It's hard to choose for yourself, but choosing for others is worse, isn't it? Have we done the right thing? It will be a thought that will haunt me for a long time. Still, I'll have to go round and see Angie now – will you phone me at the surgery to let me know how you get on with the care placement?'

A crisis point has been reached. Angie may have to go into hospital, and Jason may have to be put, at least temporarily, into foster care. For the first time in Angie's story the professional helpers involved find themselves explicitly discussing a moral question. What should be done? Should we separate mother and child? Should we keep them together and risk injury to the child? This is far from the first moral question in Angie's story, but this one must be answered. The options must be examined in the light of the information available. The different professional workers, who have tried to help Angie, must now share their experience and come to some agreed conclusion. Delay could prove fatal and the wrong decision could cause much unhappiness for Angie and her child.

The atmosphere in the case conference seemed to have been friendly and co-operative, with an absence of the professional rivalry and dogmatism which can sometimes mar such discussions. Yet to some its outcome was less than satisfactory. Probably much of the time the argument had tended to go round in circles, with the more strong-minded participants merely re-iterating their views. Certainly the decision which was reached left some people feeling apprehensive and uneasy, unsure about whether they were doing all that could be done for Angie and her baby. In situations with such a stark dilemma it is pointless to expect a simple solution. Yet perhaps the conclusion of the case conference would have seemed better to all concerned if the issues had been discussed more carefully and logically than they apparently were.

People who take decisions of this kind need to learn how to argue rationally about moral issues, and yet such skills are not at present a part of the standard training of doctors, nurses or social workers. It is hardly surprising, then, that the standard of reasoning on such case conferences is often quite low. Yet there is nothing so mysterious about the nature of moral reasoning. In form, it is the same as reasoning in any other fields – a bad argument is a bad argument, whether it is one about scientific data, treatment options or moral choices. People are more nervous about moral arguments because the assumptions from which they begin are often grounded on strong personal conviction. But (as we shall see) the moral assumptions underlying medical ethics are rarely in dispute. It is in the application of these assumptions to specific cases that the disputes arise, but it is precisely here that an analysis of reasoning is needed.

We can see the logical features of the discussion of Angie and her baby by paying attention to two ingredients of the arguments which the participants were employing:

(i) The concepts they were using in describing the problem;
(ii) The reasons which they gave to justify their conclusion.

In everyday discussion these features are not normally noticed. People simply argue their case, and we are either convinced or not convinced, without thinking much about why. But when there is genuine disagreement about the right decision, it becomes essential to look critically at the logic of people's arguments. Sometimes the argument which convinces us is far from the most rational. Faulty arguments can be remarkably persuasive, if we do not recognize their weaknesses.

Clarifying Concepts

The most obvious feature of the case conference was probably the extent to which people *agreed* with one another. Everyone wanted to avoid causing harm to Angie and her baby. Everyone agreed that Angie was showing increasing signs of disturbance, which indicated the need for some kind of psychiatric help. No one wanted to separate mother and child unless this was really necessary. Everyone wanted to stop things getting worse, fearing that, unless help was given soon, Jason could be seriously, even fatally, assaulted. It was clear that all the case conference participants shared certain common moral aims: averting pain and alleviating suffering; preventing premature death; promoting health in mother and child. Such aims are widely accepted, especially amongst people whose profession is caring for the sick and disadvantaged.[1] The problem is how to put these aims into practice in the specific decisions to be taken.

The participants in the case conference found that what they thought they held in common was in fact open to wide variations in interpretation. The *language* might be the same, but the *concepts* to which the words in the language were referring were quite different. Abercrombie, in a study of how medical students understood the word 'normal', discovered at least six different areas of meaning referred to by her sample.[2] We can expect just as much variation in value-laden terms like 'suffering' and 'health'.

Thus in the case conference there would be a wide variation in the way the different professions understood the danger of harm to Jason. The social worker may have associated 'harm' with the many emotionally deprived children he had worked with, and so opposed the separation of Jason and Angie. The police representative, on the other hand, would think of 'grievous bodily harm' and have a mental picture of the horrifying examples of child battering he had seen in the course of his police duty. The psychiatrist may have shared elements of both these thoughts. He would have encountered cases of *post partum* depression and could imagine the effect on Angie of separation from her baby, but he also, knowing the irrationality and unpredictability of the untreated depressed person's behaviour, might fear for Jason's safety.

It is pointless to argue that there is just one correct meaning for a word like 'harm', which all the participants should have used. Instead we must observe that people have certain *model cases* derived from their own experience which influence their use of such concepts.[3] Discussion will be improved if we ask people to describe what to them would be a clear case of harm as they understand it. This provides model cases which illustrate the wide range of usage which leads to disagreement. Of course, they may still disagree with each other after this clarification has been done, but there is the possibility that they will gain a fuller understanding of the situation under discussion and the least we can hope for is a better understanding of why they disagreed.

Let us imagine how the case conference might have proceeded if the participants had been aware of such conceptual ambiguities:

Social Worker: Really it would be a great mistake to take Jason into care. At this stage in his development that could cause irreparable harm.

Policeman: You talk of 'irreparable harm'! You should see some of the cases I've had to deal with: bruises, broken limbs, cigarette burns – that's harm for you.

Social Worker: Yes, I know what you mean. These cases are appalling – and it's the last thing I'd want to happen with Angie and Jason, but I'm also thinking of the kids who'll likely cross your path later in life anyway. Someone puts them into care, thinking they were best away from their own parents, and they land up emotionally insecure for the rest of their lives. That's what *I* mean by causing Jason irreparable harm.

General Practitioner: I'm sure we'd all agree that we don't want Jason either physically assaulted *or* emotionally crippled. The point is, which is the greater risk? I wonder what the psychiatrist thinks. Can Angie be trusted with Jason in her present mental state?

Psychiatrist: I'm afraid I can't give you a straight answer to that. We don't know an awful lot about *post partum* depression yet, and there are complicating factors in Angie's case – the absent boyfriend, the difficult mum and so on. Anyway, the more you see of child abuse the more you realize how little it correlates neatly with psychiatric disorder. It seems that *any* parent can get really violent at times, given a set of circumstances we really can't predict very accurately. But I'll give you a straight answer on one point. If we don't do something quickly about Angie's depression she might harm herself, and could continue to neglect the baby rather than actually assaulting him.

I'd favour a short period in hospital without the baby. I doubt if that would be particularly harmful to Jason, provided the fostering is good.

Social Worker: I still feel you're all underestimating the effects of a separation which Jason will feel, but can't possibly understand. Physical abuse is so obvious that we fear it far more than emotional trauma, but who's to say it's a worse pain?

We see all the participants in this imaginary discussion trying to clarify what they mean by 'harm' in Jason's case. The policeman and the social worker offer the model cases which are influencing their uses of the concept and this allows the general practitioner to summarize the difference as 'physical assault' versus 'emotional crippling'. The subsequent comments by the psychiatrist and the social worker reveal that this contrast is a little too simple. Angie might harm her baby by neglect, not actual assault, and a separation need not be so 'crippling', in the psychiatrist's professional opinion. The final remarks by the social worker uncover the extensive ambiguities in the concept of harm, especially when it is applied to a baby's emotional health.

The discussion also illustrates two additional ways of clarifying concepts. We can look for cases where a crucial difference means that despite first appearances the concept does not apply (*contrary cases*). An example would be the psychiatrist's reference to a *short* separation with *good* fostering, which would therefore not be harmful. We can also look for cases where we are genuinely uncertain about whether the concept applies (*borderline cases*). An example here would be the social worker's final comment on how difficult it is to estimate emotional damage in a baby. This all helps the participants to reflect upon their concept of harm and their reasons for taking a particular stance towards the case. We notice that the jargon we have been using to describe the conceptual clarification (model cases, contrary cases, etc.) need not be mentioned in the discussion itself, but the careful thinking described by the jargon is essential, as the following imaginary alternative version of the discussion illustrates:

Policeman: The girl's a head case that's obvious. She'll batter that kid, I'll guarantee. People like that shouldn't be allowed to have children. Take the baby into care, I'd say.
Social Worker: Haven't you read Bowlby? All you're doing is passing on the emotional trauma to Jason, who'll pass it to the next generation.
General Practitioner: Let's get the medical view of this. Is she clinically depressed? That's the point. What's your opinion, Doctor?
Psychiatrist: Really hospitalization is the only answer. There's no doubt this is a *post partum* depression which is very amenable to a combination of ECT and anti-depressants. Why hesitate? – any delay could mean a worsening of the condition. She can't care for the child the way she is, so let's admit her, as quickly as possible.
Social Worker: Oh, I give up. I warn you, I'll oppose this all the way down the line. It's a child's happiness that's at stake, *and* a mother's rights!

In this version of the discussion no one is willing to listen to anyone else. Their contributions fail to connect because they simply do not share a common language, and no attempt is made to discover one. Of course each participant thinks that what he or she is saying is perfectly clear and obvious, but that is because they have not troubled to question the assumptions from which they are arguing. The conceptual worlds of the policeman, the social worker and the two doctors are not open to examination – the members of their own profession understand them perfectly well! There are, in addition, a number of invalid methods of reasoning in each person's argument, but we shall delay discussion of these until the basic structure of all forms of argument has been explained.

Giving Reasons

Let us suppose that the discussion of Angie's case has proceeded in the open and reasonable manner of the first imaginary version, that all the participants have had a chance to clarify their own views and gain an understanding of alternative ones. Sooner or later the conference will have to come to a decision, ideally one in which all the members have a share, though this may not always be achieved. How is such a decision reached?

Here is how the discussion might proceed:

Chairman: Well, we've given this case a pretty good airing. Any further points anyone wishes to make? . . . No? Right, we've heard the various opinions on Angie Carter's current situation, what do you propose we do?

Psychiatrist: I hesitate to speak first, since I've only met the patient once, but I think I'd press for in-patient treatment as soon as possible, with the baby in foster care.

Social Worker: Well, I'm not happy with that. Can't the GP get her on to antidepressants while we continue with regular home visits? Finding a suitable place for Jason wouldn't be easy – and Angie is just beginning to develop a bond with him.

General Practitioner: No, that won't wash. Our experience with Angie over medication isn't good. Frankly I don't think she'd keep on with the tablets. We've also already had one overdose attempt – and I don't fancy the responsibility, if she *does* really injure Jason.

Policeman: I'm for erring on the safe side too. I see the point about separation and all that, but we've had enough warning signs to justify direct action here for the baby's safety.

Chairman: Well, what's it to be? Sounds like the majority favour hospital admission for Angie. Is that correct?

Health Visitor: No. I favour Mr Jackson's solution. It's a shame to take Jason away, when Angie's just learning to cope quite well.

Chairman: Well, I'd rather not put this to a vote or anything like that. Let's go over the various arguments again . . .

Let us do the chairman's job for him, but in a way he would not normally adopt. Ordinary language leaves many features of arguments merely implied or half-stated. Can we discover the logical structure of the opposing arguments of pyschiatrist and social worker by teasing out these features? Here we shall follow the analysis of arguments suggested by Toulmin *et al.* in *An Introduction to Reasoning.*[4]

We begin by stating the recommendations which the psychiatrist and social worker want the case conference to adopt. These are described as *claims* (C):

PSYCHIATRIST

C(laim)

Angie should be admitted to hospital for treatment without Jason

SOCIAL WORKER

C(laim)

Angie should be treated at home and not separated from Jason

Each of these claims rests on certain *grounds* (G) which the participants have stated earlier and so do not trouble to repeat. We can add them as follows:

PSYCHIATRIST

G(rounds) ⟶ C(laim)

Angie has a *post partum* depression	So, she should be admitted to hospital for treatment without Jason

SOCIAL WORKER

G(rounds) ⟶ C(laim)

There is a bond developing between Angie and Jason	So, Angie should be treated at home and not separated from Jason

Perhaps it seems rather pedantic to fill in this detail, but it helps us to see precisely on what each person's claim is based. Often this in itself is enough to question the claim, since the grounds stated may be open to dispute or insufficient to establish the claim. However, in the case of Angie everyone agrees that there is psychiatric disturbance and that there exists a developing bond between her and Jason. We might, however, press both the psychiatrist and the social worker to convince us that the grounds they offer really do establish the claim. This is called asking for a *warrant* (W), and, if that does not seem a self-evident justification, we can then ask for their *backing* (B) for this warrant. The next diagram summarizes how this might be done.

PSYCHIATRIST

G ──────────────────▶ C

Angie has a *post partum* depression

So, she should be admitted to hospital for treatment without Jason

W(arrant)
Because only hospitalization is effective for such cases

B(acking)
As is shown by various studies of treatment for this illness

SOCIAL WORKER

G ──────────────────▶ C

There is a bond developing between Angie and Jason

So, Angie should be treated at home and not separated from Jason

W(arrant)
Because separation causes emotional trauma

B(acking)
As is shown by studies of the effects of maternal deprivation

At this stage in the argument the rival claims seem to be evenly matched. No one questions the grounds on which the claims are based and each claim is backed up, not just by a personal opinion, but by an appeal to research studies which give authority to the warrant. Have we then got a case of an irresistible force meeting an immovable object? Not necessarily. It depends on how strongly each claim is being asserted (Is it being put forward as necessarily so, or only probably so?); and on whether there are certain circumstances in which the claim would not hold. We describe the former as the *modality* (M) of the claim and the latter the *rebuttal* (R) of the claim. Both the psychiatrist and the social worker have been quite flexible and undogmatic in their assertions, so we may suppose that they would regard their claims as merely probable, not absolutely certain, and that they could imagine circumstances which might invalidate the claim. The full structure of each argument, adding these features, can now be laid out as follows:

PSYCHIATRIST

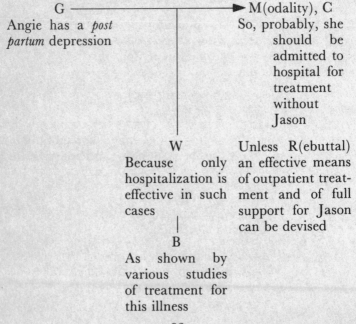

G

Angie has a *post partum* depression

M(odality), C

So, probably, she should be admitted to hospital for treatment without Jason

W

Because only hospitalization is effective in such cases

Unless R(ebuttal) an effective means of outpatient treatment and of full support for Jason can be devised

B

As shown by various studies of treatment for this illness

SOCIAL WORKER

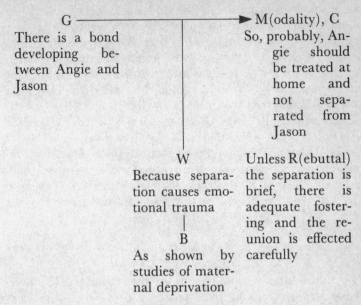

G ─────────────► M(odality), C

There is a bond developing between Angie and Jason

So, probably, Angie should be treated at home and not separated from Jason

W
Because separation causes emotional trauma
|
B
As shown by studies of maternal deprivation

Unless R(ebuttal) the separation is brief, there is adequate fostering and the reunion is effected carefully

The reader may feel that it has taken a long time to reach the position already established several pages back! But it is important to see the structure of the two arguments. The following points should be noted:

(1) By asking for warrants, backing and modality we put ourselves in a better position to assess the strength of a claim. We can imagine, for example, that the research studies quoted as backing might be questioned by some members of the group and alternative studies quoted. This would help to clarify how reliable the claim is and to establish its degree of probability.

(2) The specification of exceptions (rebuttals) is particularly important, since this opens a way to compromise. In the restatement of the claims by psychiatrist and social worker we find a basis for a responsible decision about Angie. The conference must decide which set of conditions is more easily met – the provision of outpatient treatment and home care, or the provision of temporary foster care, a brief period in hospital and support when Jason returns to Angie. If they

cannot guarantee to meet either set of conditions then they have not found a way out of the dilemma.

As with the technical language about conceptual clarification, it is not being suggested that the jargon of claims, grounds, warrants, etc., should be imported into case conference discussions. The point is rather that the style of thinking which the language describes should be adopted, by asking questions like: 'What's your basis for that view?' 'How definite is that connection?' 'Are there exceptions to this? Can you spell them out?' Such demands for a logical structure to arguments become especially important when people are using (deliberately or merely through laziness) invalid methods for establishing a claim. The logician's name for these is 'fallacies', but we prefer the less dignified description, 'dirty tricks'.

Dirty Tricks

In our alternative version of the case discussion (p. 88 above) the participants took up fixed positions from which they proceeded to launch attacks on each other. We have noted already that in such an atmosphere people will not be prepared to reflect on the concepts they are using (e.g. the policeman's use of 'head case', the social worker's reference to 'emotional trauma', the GP's 'medical view' and the psychiatrist's concept of 'amenable to treatment'). The participants were using words for their emotional force, rather than considering whether the descriptions they were offering actually fitted the situation under discussion. In addition, they failed to see that the words that carry force for them do not work in the same way for others. The policeman was no more impressed by the doctor's phrase 'medical view' than the doctor was with the policeman's use of 'head case'. But as well as failing to clarify the concepts they were using, all the participants in this version of the case discussion used a number of 'dirty tricks' to try to win the argument. Their claims might have convinced some people, easily moved by rhetoric, but they were all sadly lacking in logical coherence.

We can uncover the fallacies in this type of arguing by considering how it could be fitted into the structure outlined above. What are the grounds, warrants and backing for the various claims? We can see that various dirty tricks were used to try to establish the claims, including (1) *begging the question*, (2) *unwarranted generalization*, (3) *appeals to authority* and (4) *evading the issue*.

(1) The policeman's comments on Angie are a good example of begging the question. His claim 'she'll batter that kid' is based on nothing stronger than his conviction that Angie is the sort who batters children. It is not clear what warrant, and still less what backing, he could give apart from his own prejudice. Thus begging the question involves prejudging an issue and then using this prejudgement in the argument. The social worker's concluding comment 'it's a child's happiness that's at stake' provides a similar example. He assumes that only *his* solution will protect Jason's happiness, and then uses this assumption to 'prove' his position!

(2) We see unwarranted generalization in the policeman's assertion: 'People like that shouldn't be allowed to have children.' He bases this claim on some extreme cases of child abuse he has encountered, generalizes this view to cover any parents who may molest their child and then (by his begging of the question) classes Angie among these parents. Similarly, the psychiatrist's confidence about hospitalization seems to be based on the successful treatment of some cases of *post partum* depression, which he then assumes must apply to *all* cases. (The modality of the psychiatrist's claim is the relevant point here. The universality of his claim is indicated by phrases like 'the only answer' and 'there's no doubt'.)

(3) The social worker uses an appeal to authority when he says to the policeman, 'Haven't you read Bowlby?' Of course, his remark is, in part, the offering of a backing from psychological research of his claim, 'On no account should we remove the baby'. But the use of Bowlby's name and the sarcastic tone of his intervention is designed to make people feel that only an illiterate fool would question his assertion! A similar ploy is used by the general practitioner. By asserting that 'the medical view' is the point, he is trying to capture the problem for the medical experts, a club of which only he and the psychiatrist are members. If his ploy works, then

anything the doctors say will carry a special authority, irrespective of its validity on logical grounds.

(4) Finally, a number of people evade the issue. One example is the collusion between the GP and the psychiatrist to treat the case only as a matter of diagnosis and treatment of illness. This allows the psychiatrist to focus on how Angie's depression can be best treated, ignoring the vital question of what is to happen to Jason in the meantime. The social worker's closing shot ('. . . *and* a mother's rights!') is another form of evasion, introducing extraneous matter to cloud the issue. No one has in fact suggested that Jason should be removed against Angie's will. Thus the question of the mother's rights has not yet arisen. Perhaps the social worker means that Angie will be subtly influenced to leave Jason and go into hospital, when really she should be free to make up her own mind. But if that is what the social worker means, he should say so. Instead he attempts to use the emotive phrase 'a mother's rights' to cast doubt on the morality of the proposal he is opposed to. It is a tactic well known to politicians, but inappropriate in a rational discussion of professional responsibilities.

These examples of begging the question, unwarranted generalization, appeals to authority and evading the issue by no means exhaust all the possibilities for fallacious argument in case conferences, but they are probably among the most frequently used, especially when moral issues are raised. Our aim in this chapter has been to alert people to the dangers of muddled thinking and fallacious reasoning and to suggest some methods of analysis which can uncover such errors. But, as we have stressed all along, we do not see the technical language of logical analysis as important in itself. It is merely an aid to clearer and more rational discussion using ordinary language. It is rather like learning to ride a bicycle. You need instructions on how to do it, but once you have got your balance, you needn't remember the instructions. We hope that moral controversies in case discussions will be more responsibly discussed if participants have had some opportunity to study these elements of logical argument. People will still disagree about what ought to be done – that can be safely predicted! If, however, disagreements are brought out into the open in this way and an atmosphere of open debate is created, there is a greater chance that the decisions reached in case conferences and other discussions between people will be based on a sense of shared responsibility.

There are however some aspects of case conferences and similar discussions which are not so readily dealt with by appeals to rational argument. Decisions are often reached through various forms of emotional manipulation, for example, the use of a forceful personality, the inappropriate exercise of authority, or the introduction of a 'hidden agenda' where the real purpose of the meeting is subverted by other goals which some of the more powerful participants are covertly seeking. Shy members of a group or people unused to expressing their thoughts in a group context may be easily intimidated by the more vocal and confident participants. A person in a senior position may make it clear by verbal or non-verbal methods that disagreement is tantamount to rebellion. A hidden agenda may spring from the career ambitions or unexpressed personal bias of an individual or rivalry between participating professions. These factors remind us that in morality reason must always be balanced by realistic emotional awareness. Angie and people like her will be helped when the professionals they encounter are not afraid to use both their rational and their emotional capacities to the full. Such a rounded approach will be needed to meet the crises which still lie ahead in Angie's story.

Exercises

1. Group Exercise: Reconstruct the case conference about Angie and Jason using role-play. The discussion should be allowed to develop freely, using the information known about Angie merely as a starting point. (As in previous role-plays, people should be encouraged to try unfamiliar roles.) Plenty of time should be left for analysis of the moral arguments used in the role-play. The role-play should be recorded if possible, or, alternatively, several people should act as observers, paying particular attention to concepts and the structure of arguments used by the different participants. (The same format can be employed with any case raising difficult choices and the setting can be changed to a ward meeting, team meeting, teaching round, etc.)

2. George Bernard Shaw (in typical style!) wrote the following in his preface to *The Doctor's Dilemma*:

Doctors are just like other Englishmen: most of them have no honor and conscience: what they commonly mistake for these is sentimentality and an intense dread of doing anything that everybody else does not do, or omitting to do anything that everybody else does. This of course does amount to a sort of working or rule-of-thumb conscience; but it means that you will do anything, good or bad, provided you get enough people to keep you in countenance by doing it also. It is the sort of conscience that makes it possible to keep order on a pirate ship, or in a troop of brigands.

Anti-English sentiment aside, to what extent is Shaw on target with regard to medical and other professional attitudes to ethics?

3. Is the following argument valid?

Every year hundreds of people die because of a lack of medical facilities in Britain, e.g. a shortage of kidney machines, inadequate casualty departments, understaffed hospital wards. But *we* elected the Government which places limits on health-service expenditure, so *we* are responsible for these people's deaths!

In assessing the argument, try to isolate claims, grounds and (implicit) warrants and backings. Would a clarification of concepts improve the argument? If it is invalid, how might the problem of responsibility for priorities in health-service expenditure be more adequately stated?

4. Identify the 'model cases' employed in the following letters to

the Press. To what extent do the model cases chosen illuminate or obscure the issue under debate?

Kidney Transplants

Sir – Since it is now possible to keep the heart beating and the blood circulating of a person decapitated by the guillotine, it is clearly no longer possible to identify the moment of death by the cessation of heart-beat.

(Letter to *The Times*, 26 February 1975)

The Unborn Child

Sir – A recent opinion poll showed a large majority in favour of the restoration of the death penalty for terrorists convicted of murder. Parliament in its infinite wisdom voted against.

An opinion poll would probably show a similar majority in favour of legal abortion. Let us hope that in the near future Parliament will again exercise its prerogative and extend the same compassion to the unborn child, repeal or reform the Abortion Act, and so remove any possible charge of hypocrisy.

(Letter to the *Daily Telegraph*, 28 December 1974)

Voluntary Euthanasia

Sir – David Forrester has missed the central point in the campaign for voluntary euthanasia (15 February). It is not in the end a matter of religious doctrine or medical ethics but rather one of personal choice in a pluralist society – as in the neighbouring areas of abortion and suicide. We are asking not for doctors or priests who disapprove of voluntary euthanasia to perform or sanction it, but only for those who approve of it to be able to make the appropriate arrangements for themselves. In our view the right to live involves the right to die when life ceases to have value; and what used to be called a Roman death may be seen as a rational death for those who wish to make up their own minds.

(Letter to *The Times*, 27 February 1975)

5. Identify and evaluate the claims contained in the following examples, paying particular attention to (explicit or implicit) warrants, backings, modality and the use, if any, of 'dirty tricks':

Unvetted Research

Pyschologists are again planning to dose the 'innately dull' with glutamic acid in an experiment to see whether it can make ESN children more mentally alive. The proposal was originally vetoed by the old Stockport Education Authority. But now the psychologists hope the new Metropolitan District Council will approve their plans ... The psychologist proposing the research discounted any ideas that these experiments should be vetted. 'This is just a quiet little research project. We are doing nothing illegal. There is no question of any outside body approving what we are doing; we are practising psychologists.'

(*Times Educational Supplement*, 10 May 1974)

Our Present Decline
As a result of the familiar confusion between legality and morality, the 1967 Abortion Act has been gradually used to change people's attitudes about what is ethically tolerable. In ten years we have reduced to a common-or-garden convenience option an action – the destruction of the unborn child – which has been regarded as morally disgusting throughout our civilization. It is, I think, one of the more obvious manifestations of our present decline, and if anybody thinks that it is politically a minor issue the answer is that politics is essentially about the value we set on human life and how we live together in society.

(Ronald Butt, *The Times*, 8 May 1975)

'We trust you'
The Counsel defending a consultant paediatrician accused of the attempted murder of a Down's syndrome baby told the jury at Leicester Crown Court they could pass a verdict telling Britain's doctors: 'We trust you'.

He said in his final address that it was a 'ghastly tragedy' that the original murder charge, which was dropped during the trial, had been made. He said 1981 would go down in the annals of criminal law as the year in which the Yorkshire Ripper and a devoted doctor had both been charged with murder.

(*The Scotsman*, 4 October 1981)

7

Conclusions

The crash made the old man rush to the window. At first he thought it must be a car on that corner again. No. Perhaps some of the boys had left school early and were up to something in the garage at the side of the block. Still, when he'd been a boy . . . Then something black came flying down past his dim right eye, and made him duck. He followed the black thing down till it hit the ground with a slap, where the broken china lay. It looked like a big book – perhaps a sort of album, but it was a bit far away down there to see without his glasses. Suddenly another crash. This time from overhead. Angie! He knew it. He had been saying to his next door neighbour only this morning that he hadn't seen her lately, and had worried that they'd taken her back into hospital. She'd said she was going regularly to some sort of day hospital, but that couldn't be right could it, as someone was up there now. Perhaps it was burglars, or maybe someone taking advantage of her. He made for the door, changed his mind, grabbed his stick, changed his mind again, and reached for the phone. He suddenly felt his age.

When Mr Jackson reached the flat, the policewoman had calmed Angie down, and the constable was helping the kind old neighbour to make some sense of the little pile of debris in the courtyard. He heaved a sigh of relief to think of Jason safely fostered in the suburbs. At least there'll be no trial by journalist, he thought. Her flat had seemed bare before, but now he realized that there was a lot in it. Or had been. Plates and bottles lay smashed on the floor, and his nose told him that Angie had been drinking. Then he realized that most of the debris was glass and paper, and most of the paper was family photographs. Angie sat in the middle of the heap, sobbing gently. The policewoman moved Angie's hand towards a mug of tea. It had grown cool before Angie would acknowledge his presence. Her hands were still clenching, tearing, destroying.

The policeman came in with a cardboard box, caught his companion's glance, and left for the kitchen.

'Is it bad, Angie?'

'That's him done for.'

Silence.

'What do you mean, Angie?'

'My dad – I've smashed all his photos and the things he gave me. In that hospital I couldn't see it but now I'm home it stares me in the face. I loved him and he loved me, but it's hung like a lead weight round my neck. I have been going down, down, and unless I tore it off, I was to drown for ever.'

She was calmer and reached out for the tea.

'Is it any better now?'

'A bit. You never knew, did you, the awfulness of loving someone so weak? That night, that night that Dad, that Dad went to hospital. . .'

Her voice trailed off.

He took a chance. 'The night he died, Angie?'

Her anger flared again.

'He should have died, but he didn't. He lived on and he's haunted me. It was me that died, really. Tony had no chance. I thought I loved him but after Dad died I didn't know any more. He worked for him you see. Dad never seemed to like him – then something else happened. I'm not sure what, but my Dad drank you see, he said it was because of Mum and her illness and all that, they used to have terrible quarrels.'

She stood and stared out of the window.

'Tony said he'd found out something terrible about Dad, something that would ruin him. I told him to get out, and I'd never believe him, whatever he said. It was after – after our first time. Our first and only time. Jason's time, I suppose, unless. . .'

This time Mr Jackson's courage deserted him. He left the 'unless' alone.

'You didn't listen to Tony?'

'No, I wouldn't believe him – and yet I did. I know what he thought about my Dad was right, because, well, it fitted. Dad and I were close, very close. There were things Tony could never know, that's why he had to go. Of course he couldn't understand. He was furious and said he'd show me. He went away in tears and must have had it out with Dad next day. Anyway, Dad came home early from work more angry than I'd ever seen him. I went to bed, Mum called the doctor, I got pills. That evening Dad tried to sort it out, but I was so angry I threw the pills at him and then, he, he fell. That's how it was. It's finished now.'

A soft knock.

'Thank you, thank you very much officer – yes, no. I won't be needing your help any more. You've been most kind.'

The incident at Angie's flat has filled in some important gaps in the jigsaw puzzle of her troubled life. In destroying the mementoes of the dead father who wouldn't die Angie has brought to the surface powerful feelings of anger and guilt, stemming from a relationship too close for comfort. We begin to see why the boyfriend remains such a shadowy figure, why there is such painful enmity between Angie and her mother, and, above all, why the night of her father's death has scarred her in a way she only half understands herself. Like so many of the clients and patients of professional agencies Angie seems to be a prisoner of the past. She is dogged by an ill-defined unhappiness, which shows itself in illness and an inability to cope. Professional helpers may offer symptom relief, may try to protect her and her baby from the damaging effects of her depression, and may even hope to assist her in gaining 'insight' into her more deep-seated problems: but eventually Angie must find her own key to freedom. Professional helpers are like crutches or other temporary aids. Their function is to offer support until the person regains strength and mobility. Angie has just begun to lay the ghosts of the past, and this is an essential prelude to living for the present and planning for the future of Jason and herself. She may well slip back again and need much more support before her inner strength develops fully, but the nourishing of that inner strength is the prime professional task.

Looking back over the story as it has unfolded, what lessons can be learned from the mistakes made by the professionals who have dealt with Angie and her family so far? And what guidelines can be given to those who would like to be more effective allies in their patients' or clients' search for health?

The Wisdom of Hindsight

The most obvious feature of Angie's story is that, before the various crises erupted, the general practitioner was the main point of contact between the family and professional health care agencies. The general practitioner service is a feature of the British Health Service often admired in other countries. It allows for a continuity of care not possible when patients have direct access to specialists, enables illness to be seen within a family setting and, because relatively minor complaints may be brought to the surgery, it assists in prevention or early detection of serious illness. Dr McVie was in this privileged position. He knew about Mrs Carter's difficult pregnancy and her breast cancer and mastectomy. His occasional visits to the home had given him a tentative impression of the family relationships. A recent visit by Angie to the surgery had alerted him to some upset which she found it impossible to talk about. His house call on Guy Fawkes night enriched these impressions. He spotted Mrs Carter's tenseness, Angie's underlying anxiety and Mr Carter's heavy drinking. Yet, because of the numerous pressures distracting his attention, Dr McVie made no use of any of this information. The reflex of pencil and prescription pad took over. He could not, of course, have predicted the dramatic events which would follow that evening, culminating in Mr Carter's fatal heart attack. Yet the fact remains that he was at that time the one person who might have seen below the surface of Mrs Carter's desperate attempts to maintain a 'respectable' façade. Angie's story might have been very different if Dr McVie had stopped to consider more carefully how he should react to her tummy ache. Perhaps he would not have been the right one to help with the deeper problems which emerged, but he was the obvious door-keeper to help from other sources.

Similar narrowness of vision is evident in many of the other professionals who deal with the Carter family. Sheila, the house-doctor, has some kind of intuition about Angie's difficulties, originating from her history-taking on the night of the heart attack, but her well-meaning efforts to act on it seem quite ineffective. There is no co-ordinated effort to help Angie during the traumatic days following Jason's birth, and to the nurses on the maternity ward she remains just a difficult patient they can't seem to cope with. Mrs Jarvis, the health visitor, is yet another professional who spots trouble, yet she seems to do little more than let her worry distract her from driving! It will take a major crisis, with police, neighbours and the mother all involved, before people start to ask fundamental questions about Angie's health and to seek longer-term solutions. The tragedy is that, because the problems have developed to this critical stage, the solutions required are more radical than anyone would really want. The unhappy sixteen-year-old schoolgirl is now a disturbed, unsupported mother with a baby in danger of neglect or injury. Doctors, social workers, health visitor and police find themselves struggling to communicate with one another about a highly complex case, which simply cannot be left to develop on its own any longer. No one relishes the responsibility of taking a decision, when all that is left is the choice of a lesser evil. Besides, the fleeting nature of everyone's contact with Angie leaves the uneasy feeling that no one can now really help her. One is left with the haunting sense of lost opportunities for a close relationship with Angie, which might have helped her over the trauma of her father's death.

Signposts

The story of Angie can be seen as a cautionary tale, which will reveal moral aspects of professional helping relationships across a wide range of situations and with patients or clients of all kinds. Thus from our 'wisdom of hindsight' about what went wrong in the attempts to help Angie we can suggest some very general principles which should govern all professional work committed to restoring or maintaining the health of others. It is not easy to think about the wider implications of relationships in the heat of the moment. Some professional encounters call for rapid decisions, especially when there is the added pressure of a full waiting-room or a heavy case-load. Thus ethical guidance has to be reasonably simple, easy to remember and of obvious practical application. For this reason we offer a number of 'signposts' which point both to goals and to pitfalls in health care. (Those who find acronyms useful will see that we aim high for 'ARCS' and avoid sitting on the 'RUMP'!) At the same time, the danger of such simplification must be noted. The signposts may help to develop some useful habits of mind (like a bias toward the autonomy of patients/clients and an insistence on reasoned argument, when disagreements occur), but many situations are so complex that they require much more reflection and debate before a responsible decision can be reached. In such complex situations a decision should be delayed whenever possible, and then the 'checklist' given in the next section of this chapter may be used to explore the moral dimensions more fully. The 'signposts' we suggest are:

AIM FOR   *A*utonomy (restoring the person's own capacities for health)

*R*ealism (about what can be changed and who can change it)

*C*omplexity (by shifting focus and viewpoint)

*S*haring (the responsibility with patient, relatives, friends and other professionals)

AVOID   *R*outines (which are kept exempt from criticism)

*U*nreasoned Solutions (based on muddled concepts)

*M*anipulation (by patients, relatives or professionals)

*P*rofessional Imperialism (i.e. seeing other professions as rivals and patients as merely passive recipients of care)

A Moral Checklist

In Chapter 1, when we first began to discuss the moral aspects of Angie's story, we referred to ethics as a minefield without maps. Although this aspect of ethics is inconvenient (though hardly as dangerous as an uncharted minefield!) it is perhaps not altogether a bad thing. Human history is full of examples of 'simple solutions' to moral problems. Usually this has resulted in some group or other being despised, exploited or liquidated, because they did not fit well into someone's master plan. It has been the task of moral philosophers throughout the ages to encourage a critique of currently accepted morality by constantly questioning the basis of ethical norms. The obvious moral answer, they have pointed out, is not always the right one, even if it is the most fashionable at the time. A critical attitude towards every system of morality is the best protection against both self-righteous moralism and the destructive influence of prejudice.

Thus any system we now suggest for checking on the morality of professional helping relationships must itself be seen as a candidate for radical critique. This is not to be seen as 'final solution' – it may not even be a very satisfactory *temporary* solution to some of the problems professionals encounter. But it represents an attempt at practical guidance, which derives (like the signposts in the previous section) from the detailed arguments of all the preceding chapters. The checklist proposed can be used by an individual who has the opportunity to reflect on some difficult case, or it might profitably be used by a group to structure discussion of the moral aspects of a case history. The checklist is intended for use by various professional groups, but to avoid the rather heavy phrase 'patient or client', the person receiving help is referred to simply as 'the patient' throughout.

(1) Has the patient been correctly identified? Who made the identification – the patient? a friend/relative? another agency? If not correctly identified, is there another person or group needing help?
(2) How does the patient see the situation?
    (a) Is the patient competent to judge?
    (b) How does this incident fit into his/her life-story?
    (c) Is more information needed before the patient's point of view can be understood?
(3) What choices are open in the situation?
    (a) for the patient
    (b) for those trying to help him/her
(4) Is anyone trying to reduce choices?
    (a) by refusing to take responsibility
    (b) by attempting to manipulate others

      (c) by assuming inappropriate control
(5) What is your understanding of the facts?
      (a) What is your viewpoint and focus?
      (b) Do others have a different viewpoint/focus?
(6) Is this a case for professional care?
      (a) How specifically can professional intervention help?
      (b) What are the limits of professional care in this case?
(7) What is the social context?
      (a) Are the social conditions a major factor? Can they be changed?
      (b) Which professional groups are involved? Are they co-operating?
      (c) What about the family?
      (d) Are there widely accepted moral norms or legal principles at stake?
(8) Any answers?
      (a) What rival claims are being made for a satisfactory solution to the problems?
      (b) What concepts underlie these claims? Can they be clarified?
      (c) How well founded are the claims? Is the reasoning behind them valid? (dirty tricks?) What rebuttals, if any, might point to a compromise?
      (d) What is your decision and how does it affect the other people involved (especially the patient)?

In Every Case

Each chapter so far has ended with exercises, to increase the reader's power and skill in one specific faculty. But for really healthy living, exercise is a total activity, intended to maintain all the faculties and to develop skill and stamina to attain new goals. In a similar way the everyday practice of morality leads to new and often unexpected developments, not just in that case, but in every case.

Why is it that it is only when things go wrong that people start to think? Postmortems have always taught doctors a great deal, but at an obvious cost. In healthier times, other ways must be used to learn, and ethical study is no exception. We must learn to anticipate and to question, before things go wrong, perhaps before even an encounter produces an 'ethical' problem at all in conventional terms. This can create a positive, anticipatory approach, based on a firm assurance that there will be problems that must be tackled, and that the most unethical response is not to notice or to fail to reflect on what we know we are seeing. 'The unexamined life is not worth living' said the irritatingly perceptive Socrates. We can choose not to make an ethical examination, just as we can omit a physical or mental assessment – but we must accept the responsibility if so.

In this positive approach we need to develop the twin facilities of sensitivity and clear thinking. There are many ways to keep sensitivity alive, and they depend greatly on circumstances. Many people find working in groups allows ideas to be challenged and motives examined in a way which is safe but stimulating – and the less 'safe' in conventional terms the group itself is, the more may be learned. Audit and evaluation can be undertaken with a group of peers, while role-play in any situation may teach the individual more about his own and his subject's life and thinking. The most challenging groups may be ones that are mixed, with other professions or with patients or clients, but it is more important to be receptive and learn to listen in the groups that already exist than to wait for 'that special learning experience' that never comes! For the individual who lacks suitable company, self-awareness remains the key to unlock everyday ethics, by allowing a response to feelings in oneself which indicate that a problem is developing that requires examination – a mounting feeling of unease, for instance, or of aggravation, or a feeling of being 'trapped' in some way. These signals are ignored at our peril. They are cues to slow down, get more information, change focus and listen to the person – the effort of attention and empathy.

Some people have no difficulties in keeping their thinking sharp, but for most it requires conscious work. Studying literature and philosophy may help, but more important is to examine that we are saying what we mean; and meaning what we say. Turning a situation, a statement or a belief on its head, or imagining roles reversed, may help to test how sharp and clear the thinking really is. 'What should I tell?' becomes 'What must he know?' or 'Why should I conceal?'

Above all we must keep moving. In a world where nothing is truly perfect, and no one is infallible, we must keep up movement, towards what declares itself as truth, not stop to guard doggedly some minor principle of the moment. In ethics, as so often in human experience, the journey matters as much as the final arrival.

Dear Dr McVie

I wonder whether you'll remember me. I hope you will, but if not you may still have the notes about the illness I had when I went into hospital and my Jason was looked after by the Council. Since I came out I've been living with my aunt over here, and it's quite difficult to get across to see you, which is why I'm writing. I feel much better now, and I think I'm well enough to look for a job – and my social worker thinks it's a good idea.

Anyway, I wonder if I could give your name to firms, as they may want a reference. Not a lot of people know me well round here, you see.

I haven't got Jason back yet, and he's still with the Council people. They look after him very well, and he's obviously quite happy there. They say it's best to get myself together first and a job might give me an interest anyway. I suppose so.

Will you be able to do this for me? Thank you and everyone in the surgery for the help they gave.

Yours sincerely

Angie Carter

P.S. I don't know how things are going to turn out for me, but here's hoping.

Recommended Reading

The following books and journals may be found helpful if the reader wishes to pursue thought and discussion along the lines we have suggested. Other titles have been mentioned in the notes.

Downie, R. S., Telfer, E., *Caring and Curing*. Methuen 1980.

Veatch, R. M., *Case Studies in Medical Ethics*. Harvard University Press 1977.

Reiser, S. J., Dyck, A. J., Curran, W. T., *Ethics in Medicine*. M.I.T. Press 1977. A collection of original articles, declarations and documents.

Campbell, A. V., *Moral Dilemmas in Medicine*, 2nd edn. Churchill Livingstone 1975.

Ramsey, P., *The Patient as Person*. Yale University Press 1970.

Kennedy, I. M., *The Unmasking of Medicine*. George Allen and Unwin 1981.

Reference Works

Walters, L. *Bibliography of Bioethics*. Published annually by Macmillan and Free Press.

Duncan, A. S., Dunstan, G. R., Welbourn, R. B., *Dictionary of Medical Ethics*, 2nd edn. Darton Longman and Todd 1981.

Reich, W. T., *Encyclopaedia of Bioethics*, 4 vols. Free Press 1978.

Specific Issues

Glover, J., *Causing Death and Saving Lives*. Penguin 1977.

Bok, S., *Lying: Moral Choice in Public and Private Life*. Quartet Books 1980.

Toulmin, S., Reike, R., Janik, A., *An Introduction to Reasoning*. Macmillan 1979.

Campbell, A. V., *Medicine, Health and Justice*: *The Problem of Priorities*. Churchill Livingstone 1978.
Wilson, J., *Thinking with Concepts*. Cambridge University Press 1963.

Journals

Hastings Centre Report (bi-monthly). Published by the Institute of Society, Ethics and the Life Sciences, 360 Broadway, Hastings-on-Hudson, NY 10706, USA.

Journal of Medical Ethics (quarterly). Published by the Society for the Study of Medical Ethics, Tavistock House North, Tavistock Square, London WC1H 9LG.

Journal of Medicine and Philosophy (quarterly). Published by the University of Chicago Press, 11030 Langley Avenue, Chicago, Illinois, USA.

Literature

Much will be learnt from novels, plays, poetry and films. The authors have indicated some of the sources which they have found helpful in the notes. Readers will probably prefer to make their own lists.

Notes and References

Chapter One: Choices

1. For a review of the statistics in British primary care see Howie, J. G. R., 'Patterns of Work' in Fry, J. (ed.), *Trends in General Practice 1979* (Royal College of General Practitioners 1979). Also see the Balint group approach to the problem discussed in Balint, E., and Norell, J. S. (eds), *Six Minutes for the Patient* (Tavistock 1973), and for international comparisons Fry, J. (ed.),*Primary Care* (Heinemann 1980).

2. A discussion of utilitarianism in relation to health care will be found in Campbell, A. V., *Moral Dilemmas in Medicine* (Churchill Livingstone 1975), ch. 3.

3. See Plant, R., 'The Greatest Happiness', *Journal of Medical Ethics*, 1975, no. 1, pp. 104–6. The references in this article are useful for a study of the arguments for and against the utilitarian approach to ethics.

4. For the Hippocratic Oath and the modern Declarations, see under the individual headings in Duncan, A.S., Dunstan, G. R., and Welbourn, R. B., *Dictionary of Medical Ethics* (Darton Longman and Todd 1981).

5. See Childress, J. F., 'Paternalism and Autonomy in Medical Decision-making' in Abernethy, V. (ed.), *Frontiers in Medical Ethics* (Bollinger 1980). A more accurate description would be 'parentalistic', but we prefer to use the more familiar term 'paternalism', even though it appears to refer only to 'fathering'.

6. 'But he who is unable to live in society, or who has no need because he is sufficient for himself must be either a beast or a God: he is no part of a state. A social instinct is implanted in all men by nature.' (*Nicomachean Ethics*, bk i, ch. 2).

7. This hazard has been most vividly portrayed by Ivan Illich in *Medical Nemesis* (Calder Boyars 1974) and *Limits to Medicine* (Penguin 1977). For a critique of Illich see Horrobin, D. F., *Medical Hubris* (Churchill Livingstone 1978).

8. Exceptions are described in the Mental Health Acts, in relation to the mentally subnormal and the severely psychiatrically disturbed patient, but in these cases other safeguards are (or should be) employed to ensure that the treatment is what the patient would have wanted, had

114

he or she been competent to decide. See Ex. 3 at the end of this chapter and Ex. 3 at the end of ch. 5.

9. For a discussion of determinism see Downie, R. S., *Journal of Medical Ethics*, 1975, no. 1, p. 49f.

Chapter Two: Facts

1. For a study of the 'lay referral system' see Friedson, E., 'Client Control and Medical Practice', *American Journal of Sociology* 1960, 65, 374–82.

2. For a summary of the problems of scientific philosophy, law and method see the relevant entries in Bullock, A., and Stallybrass, O., *The Fontana Dictionary of Modern Thought* (Fontana/Collins 1977). One of Sir Karl Popper's important contributions has been to point out that theories or facts are scientific not because they are verifiable but in so far as they are falsifiable or refutable. See Popper, K. R., *The Logic of Scientific Discovery* (Hutchinson 1959).

3. The explanatory force of scientific theory may not survive changes in scale. The classical principles that enabled Newton to explain motion successfully on one scale were called into question by Einstein when different orders of magnitude were involved. Further examples can be found in Thompson, D'A. W., *On Growth and Form* (Cambridge University Press 1966). There is an interesting analogy here with the limits of use of ethical principles: 'The mistake that people make is, they think a moral principle is indefinitely extendable, that it holds good for any situation . . .' as one of the philosophers says in the second of the two plays, Stoppard, T., *Every Good Boy Deserves a Favour* and *Professional Foul* (Faber and Faber 1979), p. 77.

4. See Fox, C., 'Training for Uncertainty' in Schwartz, H. D., and Kart, C. S., (eds), *Dominant Issues in Medical Sociology* (Addison-Wesley Publishing Company 1978). It has also been observed that homeless people in a big city often return to the railway station or bus terminus through which they first entered the city.

5. See Elstein, A. S., Shulman, L. S., and Sprafka, S. A., *Medical Problem Solving* (Harvard University Press 1978). Both this and the subsequent chapter will be further illuminated by Wulff, R., *Rational Diagnosis and Treatment* (Blackwell Scientific Publications 1976).

Chapter Three: Cases

1. Statements made by clinical medical students at seminars attended by the authors.

2. Quoted by Marinker, M., in 'Why make people patients?' *Journal of Medical Ethics*, 1975, no. 1, pp. 81–4.

3. Extract from 'How the Poor Die' in Orwell, G., *Collected Essays, Journalism and Letters*, vol. iv (Penguin 1970). This volume also includes some moving letters which Orwell wrote about his last illness.

4. This phrase implies that in a research project involving comparisons of treatments (usually drugs) neither the patient nor the doctor knows at that time which of the treatments being tested is being used. This may involve the use of a placebo. A sane view of applied research in

the health services is Cochrane, A. L., *Effectiveness and Efficiency* (Nuffield Provisional Hospitals Trust 1972).

5. See Exercises at the end of this chapter.

6. Reported by Cartwright, A., in *Social Class Variations in Health Care and in the Nature of General Practitioner Consultations* (London Institute for Social Studies in Medical Care 1975). In this document she reports that tape-recorded consultations between doctors and middle-class patients averaged 6·2 minutes, whereas those with working-class patients averaged 4·7 minutes.

7. This is a phrase introduced by Tudor Hart, J., in 'The Inverse Care Law', *Lancet* 1971, I, 405–12. In this article he argues that medical care is least easily obtained in those areas and by those pateints who need it most.

8. See Mechanic, D., *Medical Sociology* (Free Press 1978).

9. For study of this as a method of decision-making see Schaff, T. J., 'Decision Rules, Types of Error, and Their Consequences in Medical Diagnosis', *Behavioural Science* 1963, no. 8, pp. 97–107.

10. Balint, M., *The Doctor, His Patient and the Illness* (Tavistock 1957).

11. For a full description of this case, and a discussion of some of its implications see 'Case Conference. Hallelujah, I'm a bum: a story from the post-christian era', *Journal of Medical Ethics* 1980, no. 6, pp. 98–100.

12. For an exposition of the 'whole person' approach see *The Future General Practitioner* (Royal College of General Practitioners 1972) and for a reassessment Marinker, M., 'Whole Person Medicine' in Cormack, J., Marinker, M., and Morrell, D. (eds), *Teaching General Practice* (Kluwer Medical 1981).

Chapter Four: Persons

1. Hardy, T., *Tess of the D'Urbervilles* (Macmillan 1963).

2. This approach to morality derives from Immanuel Kant's account of the moral law as treating others as 'ends in themselves and not mere means'. For a modern version of this approach see Downie, R. S., and Telfer, E., *Respect for Persons* (Allen and Unwin 1969), and for its limits, Glover, J., *Causing Death and Saving Lives* (Penguin 1977). .

3. In Act One of Miller, A., *Death of a Salesman* (Penguin 1961).

4. Orwell, G., *Down and Out in Paris and London* (Penguin 1966).

5. The final lines of Auden, W. H., 'Musée des Beaux Arts', *Collected Shorter Poems 1927–1957* (Faber and Faber 1966). Icarus was the son of Daedalus. He flew with his father from Crete, but went too near the sun. The wax holding his wings melted, and he fell to his death in the sea. The painting of this scene is by Pieter Brueghel (*c.* 1525–69).

6. See Sheehy, G., *Passages* (Bantam Books 1977). For a good summary of the researched connections between life events and physical and mental illness see Hill, P., Murray, R., and Thorley, A. (eds)., *Essentials of Postgraduate Psychiatry* (Academic Press 1979).

7. Writing one's own 'Life Story Books' has become a useful technique in social work – see Lightbown, C., *Adoption and Fostering*, 1979, 3, 9–15, as an example from child care.

8. The phrase is from Eliot, T. S., 'Whispers of Immortality', *Collected Poems* 1909–1962 (Faber and Faber 1974).

Chapter Five: Relations
1. The Donne quotation is from *Devotions upon Emergent Occasions,* no. xvii (1623) and that of J. P. Satre from *Huis clos*, sc. 5.
2. Larkin, Philip, 'This Be the Verse', *High Windows* (Faber and Faber 1974), p. 30. The poet concludes that it is best to stop the cycle by not having children: but compare his most tender poem to Sally Amis, 'Born Yesterday' in *The Less Deceived* (Marvell Press 1977).
3. Case collected by the authors.
4. The pattern would probably be formulated as a bi-polar or manic-depressive puerperal psychosis.
5. See Lesser, A. H., *Journal of Medical Ethics*, 1975, no. 1, pp. 193–5 for a discussion of authority using Max Weber's categories 'legal-rational', 'charismatic' and 'traditional', which are similar to the ones we have used.
6. Case collected by the authors.
7. Case collected by the authors.
8. Games seen as a serious explanation of human interaction are best known through Berne, E., *Games People Play* (Penguin 1964), but have been brilliantly developed for application in the medical field in Browne, K., and Freeling, P., *The Doctor–Patient Relationship* (Livingstone 1967). The game in the text is our own.
9. Derived from the authors' training experience.

Chapter Six: Reasons
1. The codes of the World Medical Association and the International Council of Nurses summarize these values.
2. Abercrombie, M. L. J., *The Anatomy of Judgement* (Penguin 1969), pp. 110–31.
3. The terminology used here, and in the subsequent discussion, is derived from Wilson, J., *Thinking with Concepts* (Cambridge University Press 1971).
4. Toulmin, S., Rieke, R., and Janik, A., *An Introduction to Reasoning* (Collier Macmillan 1979).

INDEX

Index

In That Case